Who's in Charge?

WHO'S IN CHARGE?

Autonomy and Mental Disorder

John W. Appel M.D.

Rutledge Books, Inc. Danbury, CT

Rutledge Books, Inc.
107 Mill Plain Road, Danbury, CT 06811
1-800-278-8533
www.rutledgebooks.com

Manufactured in the United States of America

Cataloging in Publication Data
Appel, John W.
Who's in Charge? Autonomy & Mental Disorder

ISBN: 1-58244-071-9

1. Mental Health. 2. Independence. 3. Identity.

Library of Congress Catalog Number: 00-100848

TABLE OF CONTENTS

Acknowledgements

At Harvard College, I studied under that awesome entomologist W.H. Wheeler; at Harvard Medical School under Walter B. Cannon, who discovered "fight-flight." At the Pennsylvania Hospital I served as a resident under Edward E. Strecker, Earl Bond and Kenneth E. Appel.

The following colleagues and friends read parts, or all, of the manuscript; and made valuable suggestions: Aaron Beck, Peter Bloom, Dexter Bullard, Philip Escoll, Walter Foulke, Theodore Friend, Elio Frattaroli, Charlton Ogburn, Richard McAdoo, George Caspar Homans, Richard Meryman, Elizabeth Pool and Eric Stake.

Above all, I thank my patients who struggled with me to find their identities.

PROLOGUE

A certain worm, a nematode, when placed on a slanting board, will crawl upward. If the board is tipped to slant in the other direction the worm will turn around and again crawl upward. The worm is negatively geotropic, genetically programmed to crawl up against gravity. All living creatures are programmed to control their behavior in ways which enhance their survival. Lorenz[1] developed "ethology," the knowledge of species specific behavior, such as crawling up against gravity as cited above. Tinbergen[2], Whorpe[3], elaborated ethology into " instinctual" behavior. E.O. Wilson[4], developed "sociobiology, "which applied this knowledge to human behavior.

Humans are genetically programmed to eat, procreate, fight or flee danger so as to enhance their survival. All human civilizations show the same patterns of behavior; all show religious behavior and dancing, which at first glance would not appear to have survival value.

So, humans are programmed to control their own behavior. To do so they must be autonomous, able to decide for themselves what they think and do and oppose control by other persons. Yet, being social animals, they must get along with other humans. Here they encounter conflict—other humans may want to control them. Such conflicts occur in all living creatures; even in ants there is tension between individual control and loyalty to the ant colony[5].

Introduction

I've written this book because, as a psychiatrist treating mentally disordered patients, I discovered something about human nature that I believe might be useful to everybody.

Everyone knows that people like to decide for themselves what to do and resent being told. For example, "You'll do what I tell you to do and you'll do it right now!" yells the exasperated father at his nine-year-old daughter." "You've made your mother cry, and your sister, too. When can I have a little peace around here?" Similarly, a forty-six-year-old patient says about her mother, "She has control of me, of course, total control. The only way I could get even would be to kill myself."

Disagreement and conflict occur constantly in human relationships, particularly intimate relationships. It is not generally known that, as my theory holds, a person's mental health, even his sanity, is at stake in such conflicts. Many people fear the responsibility incurred by deciding for themselves and prefer to let others decide for them. Submitting endlessly to control by others ultimately leads to mental disorder, according to my theory. Deciding for one's self maintains mental health. One of the more difficult actions a person takes in his daily life is to oppose someone he loves and depends on. Doing so annoys and may alienate the loved one. My theory shows that autonomy is necessary to both preserve mental health and love.

Many people in our culture are confused about responsibility at present. Who is responsible for the consequences of smoking, for example? The individual who smokes? Or the tobacco companies who make, advertise and sell cigarettes? Who is responsible for the deaths of schoolmates and teachers killed by the gunshots of children? The children who pull the trigger? The schools? The parents of the children? Society? What is the proper responsibility of government? What is the responsibility of the governed? Self reliance is an American tradition. To what extent should an individual be held responsible for his own welfare and the consequences of his actions?

As a psychiatrist I became interested in autonomy and the responsibility it incurs while treating psychoses, thirty-four cases over the course of years. These patients are not autonomous, not responsible; rather they are helpless, controlled by others, "the voices," TV, or passing strangers. And they are angry, furious at the people they love and depend on, usually family members, whom they accuse of dominating and controlling them. They are "mad" in both senses of the word—angry and insane. In treatment, finding ways to help them gain autonomy cured them.

The question arises: What is autonomy? Why is it so important?

This book is an answer. The book is not merely about the treatment of psychoses. It deals with the problems of responsibility in everyday life for everybody. It describes the battle for autonomy, how it is won or lost in childhood, how the conflict plays out in adulthood. The book suggests ways of dealing more effectively with the dynamics of responsibility, interacting with other people, and of avoiding mental disorder in one's self.

The book is written for professionals and general readers, for anyone interested in human behavior. In this book I present examples of the evidence—segments of three clinical cases in verbatim detail. I show how autonomy enables a person both to resolve conflicts over control, yet preserve mental health. I show how autonomy is normally developed, or not developed, and illustrate how it can be developed in treatment.

In medicine, study of the abnormal leads to understanding of the normal. For example, liver function is revealed by studying liver disease. Study of psychogenic mental disorder shows the normal function of the human brain, which is to control behavior.

Study of neuroses, personality disorders, addictions, and other relatively minor disorders has yielded much knowledge and theory, particularly psychoanalytic theory, of human behavior. However, unlike psychotics, these patients are relatively able to control their behavior. As a result psychoanalytic hypotheses have been focused on motives, meanings and feelings.

On the other hand, a physician faced with a psychotic patient focuses on what the patient does or may do, rather than on his motives, whys and wherefores. Can the patient tell you who he is or where he is? Can he find his way home? Or will he get lost? Does he follow cultural social cues? Is he weird? Is he suicidal or homicidal? If he cannot control himself, can his family control him—or her? As a practical matter, can the physician let the patient leave his office unattended, or must he lock his office door so the patient can't get out? Of course, the physician is interested, secondarily, in motives as clues to how the patient will act.

Thus the theory proposed in this book, though it includes psycho-dynamics, is primarily behavioral. It is objective—externally observable, verifiable and measurable. Conventional psychoanalysis is subjective, dealing primarily with the dynamics of internal conflict and motives. Observation and measurement of subjective experience is difficult, if not impossible. My theory deals with conflict between the self and other individuals. Despite constant attempts, measurable criteria for psychopathology have not been found and are much needed to demonstrate degrees of disability and effectiveness of treatment.

My theory of autonomy applies not only to keeping a person sane, but also to preventing and treating less disabling disorders, which are also rooted in issues of control—neuroses, personality disorders, addictions, and most other disorders listed in the official categories of mental disorder, D.S.M. III and IV[6].

Although developed psychologically, the theory turned out to have a physiological basis. The thrust of the book is psychological—psychiatric. Physiological aspects are stated, but elaborated only briefly and supported by references to the literature, rather than direct clinical evidence, as is done with the psychological theory.

In traditional psychoanalysis, autonomy is important, but is only one of many motives in the patient's internal conflicts. My theory defines autonomy differently, as action in the concrete world—the ability to cause an effect in others. People affect other people by what they do while interacting, not by their motives.

Compared to conventional theories, these ideas have explained, to me, certain clinical observations more successfully, and have provided more effective means of treating mental disorders. My theory of autonomy works—patients get well. More important it demonstrates the advantages as well as disadvantages of taking responsibility for one's actions and welfare..

In writing this book I did not thoroughly integrate my theory with current literature. I depended on my clinical evidence. Examples, particularly three cases, are explored in detail in three chapters. All names have been changed to protect privacy.

My theory may appear simplistic, may seem too concerned with familiar manifest behavior, unaware of unconscious motivation and of complexities and multi-determinations. The reader might keep in mind that just because a concept is simple does not mean it is false: a punch in the nose is simply a punch in the nose, a kiss is a kiss.

Or readers will ask, so what else is new? Psychoanalysis and psychiatry have accepted autonomy as central. Everyone knows that self-reliance is desirable. I have taken the concept to a radically new dimension. New is that social interaction involves conflict between internal and external control and that autonomy is necessary for mental health. New to treatment is that the physician rewards his patient's autonomous behavior in the therapeutic interaction. Doing so develops and maintains the patient's autonomy. New is that the patient's brain reward system, an anatomical-physiological structure, can be used for this purpose.

In the terminology which follows, the word ego is used to denote various functions and also the sense of identity, the "I" or "me." Use of the word "mother" is generic. It refers to the primary caretaker, usually a mother, with whom the child's patterns of social interaction ordinarily develop during the years of intense dependence . I am not denying the role of the father, siblings, or friends. Use of the word "he" has no gender significance, and is used merely to avoid the awkward "he/she."

CHAPTER ONE

AUTONOMY AND PSYCHOSIS

The reader of this page could have a nervous "breakdown," could even become psychotic, insane. The reader may think this idea is preposterous. He doesn't believe it. He takes it for granted that he is perfectly stable. The ordinary cultural assumption is that a normal person's mental health is strong, easily able to withstand the stresses or ordinary living and therefore is not at risk. This is not true. A person's mental health is vulnerable to domination by other people, repeated failure, rejection, scorn. Most people have only a vague definition of mental health. To them mental disorder is a weird, frightening craziness that, thank goodness, has nothing to do with them. It is something that happens only to "neurotics." My theory suggests that normal people are also vulnerable, all people have a breaking point, all have the same problems as those who have broken down, only less severe.

People suffer the stresses of failures at work, rejection, criticism, domination—and are angered and frightened. If the stresses are sufficiently severe and prolonged, they cause a mental breakdown. This means that if exposed to extreme abnormal stress any normal man may break down mentally. This had not been known to psychiatry, or to anyone, until World War II when Gilbert Beebe, Ph.D., a statistician, and I, a psychiatrist, published a study[7] showing that the continual danger of injury, death—and hearing "them shells"—seeing men wounded and killed, hearing screams, for a definite period of time—240 aggregate days—to be exact—of front-line infantry combat, cause "combat fatigue" in all those exposed. Even combat veterans, sergeants with multiple stripes for combat service and decorations developed startle, tremors, confusion and other symptoms of incapacitating psychiatric disorder.

A further example of a normal man's vulnerability to extreme stress is shown dramatically by sensory-deprivation experiments in which a person is immersed, blindfold in a tank of water at body temperature. All external stimuli are removed. In the darkness there is no vision, sound or touch—and no possibility of doing anything to change the environment. Mental function rapidly breaks down; anxiety mounts; the person becomes confused, disoriented and after an hour or so develops illusions and even delusions. Removed from the tank and restored to sights and sounds and interaction with other people, mental function promptly returns.[8]

Solitary confinement in prisons results in similar symptoms, though not as severe since some interaction occurs. A different kind of isolation occurs in patients suffering from schizophrenia and other severe mental disorders. Here the symptoms develop because these patients are unable to interact with other people. They are in the psychological equivalent of an isolation tank, private, self induced. Here there is no possibility of emerging. The loneliness is unrelieved.

It is clear a person requires constant interaction with his environment to stay sane. Breathing to maintain oxygenation is a similar interaction with the non-social environment.

So anyone can become mentally disordered under abnormal stress. Under normal, everyday stress, only abnormal people breakdown. "Weakness" is not necessary to explain their vulnerability. The three patients presented here had been rendered abnormal—vulnerable—by parents who dominated them, who didn't "listen," and who dismissed their thinking, One patient broke down because he could not handle rebellious subordinates in his job, another patient broke down because she could not get along with other people, she thought everybody "hated" her. Another young woman could not handle boy friends. These stresses are normally successfully met by most people.

Fortunately, any person responds to positive experience, successes of one kind or another, to signs of respect or affection. In fact much of human experience represents the ups and downs of his ego and attempts to build up and defend it. In the same way that physical pain indicates injury to the body, any threat or injury to the ego is signaled by psychological pain—anxiety, low self esteem. hurt feelings, or shame. These threats evoke anger and fear, which become the energy to destroy or to escape the danger—the so-called "fight-flight" mechanism.[9]

Psychotic patients are not autonomous, rather they are helpless, unable to control their behavior. Their parents had overcontrolled them: what to think, what and how much to eat, who to play with and so on. The patient's attempt to make one's own decisions had not been rewarded. They remained helpless and dependent. Mental breakdown was the result. The patient's rage represented their will to live, to exist and so to take control of what they did—the drive for autonomy. Rewarding decision making in therapeutic interaction develops autonomy and cures these patients

Conventional psychoanalysis—interpreting dreams, for example is of limited value treating the acute phase of psychosis. Treating such patients, the physician is more concerned with what they will do. He is less concerned with their motives.

People affect each other by what they do, not by their motives. Finding new ways to restore the patient's autonomy, their ability to take control of their actions, is effective. The patients get well, thereby confirming the necessity for autonomy. Current theory specifies that the patient and analyst interact with each other. However I define interact differently. I emphasize the "act" element of interact. The analyst does things to the patient and conversely the patient does things to the analyst.

All theories emphasize "listening" to patients. However current theory sees listening as passive, essentially a sensory experience by the clinician. My theory sees "listening" as active. interactive, transactional, behavioral, using all the vast number of complex elements of social interaction. And the physician in particular rewards the patient's behavior, much as a mother does her child. Details of the treatment method used will be presented in Chapter Seven.

In patients suffering from less severe types of mental disorder—and in ordinary people every day—the strugggle for autonomy is ubiquitous. All animals, including humans, are genetically programmed to control their behavior to survive and reproduce.

Normal adults are autonomous, they control their thinking and behavior and can oppose control by other people. They recognize intuitively that the ubiquitous conflicts between autonomy and love in their personal lives endanger identity. They seek means of resolving these conflicts without losing the love of the other person or losing their "sanity." Husbands and wives stay relatively calm—sane—when arguing with each other. Parents deal with the "terrible twos," and with rebellion in their adolescents. Tyrants, domestic or political, are feared and hated. "Freedom" interests everybody, and with good reason—the stakes are high.

The theory of autonomy presented here is new to psychiatric and psychoanalytic thought. Psychoanalysis has no theory of action. Indices of text books of psychoanalysis, psychiatry or psychology scarcely mention the words "autonomy," or "independence". As Shapiro[10] has said the concept of autonomy has not been integrated into psychoanalysis, psychiatry or psychology. The concept of interaction between people was introduced to psychiatry by Harry Stack Sullivan[11] and had led to interpersonal, two-person psychoanalysis, "attachment" theory, inter-subjective analysis, object-relations theory. In recent years words containing the syllable "act" have appeared in psychoanalytic literature with increasing frequency. However, none of these writers present my theory of autonomy and its relation to Mental Disorder.

The theory I suggest focuses on "control" of behavior. The word "control" is still new to psychoanalysis. It is not even mentioned in the standard compendium of Terms and Concepts of the American Psychoanalytic Association.[12] The extensive literature on the psychotherapy of Schizophrenia, including writings of authorities such as Frieda Fromm-Reichman[13], Arieti[14] does not present the role of autonomy. The word power and "helplessness" is new. "Control" does exist in the literature of psychology and of social work—including the relation to identity. But no connection is made to autonomy or mental disorder.

In fiction the relation of autonomy to sanity has long been a favorite theme. For example in the play, "Separate Tables", by Terrance Rattigan[15], a grown daughter saves her sanity when she refused, for the first time in her life, to obey a demand from her dominating mother. In the novel, "The Late George Apley," by John P. Marquand[16] a lover says, "If I depend on you too much, there will be no more me."

Thinkers in all disciplines—psychiatry, philosophy, and

social science—have long been interested in human autonomy. Yet none of these writers offer my suggestion that social interaction involves conflict for control. Freud positioned autonomy of the ego from the id, superego, and external reality. Alexander[17] said, "the ego has been less studied and understood and published than the id. This is because psychoanalysis started with interest in the abnormal, second we have less knowledge of the ego...Much of it was already a matter of common sense. Common sense and rational behavior are always with us and are taken for granted but not methodically described. To explain them appears an elaboration of the obvious." Erik Erikson[18] in 1950 was the first to develop the concept of autonomy. Heinz Kohut[19] wrote about the development and structure of the self. Margaret S. Mahler[20] gave a beautiful description of the infant's individuation and separation from the mother. Jean Piaget[21] described stages of cognitive development and in "Cognitive Science," Howard Gardner[22] dealt with decision making. John Searles[23] wrote a summary of the subject from a philosophical viewpoint.

David Shapiro[op.cit 20] gave the most direct and clear description of autonomy and its role in mental health, particularly as related to Compulsive Personality. In 1993 Leo Rangell[24] proposed a theory of action in psychoanalysis which included a description of choice, conflict and ego decision-making. Authorities have written specifically about autonomy: Fairbairn[25], Guntrip[26], Bowlby[27], Hartmann[28], Holt[29], Lichtenstein[30], Huizenga[31], Givelber[32], Schafer[33], Sutherland[34]. More recently, 1997, Stephen M. Mitchell[35] wrote "The Influence of Autonomy in Psychoanalysis" which comes the closest, but is far short of my theory.

None of these writers describe the conflict between autonomy, attachment and mental disorder.

Chapter Two
Developing Identity

"To be is to do" — Plato

"There are two feelings, pleasure and pain, which affect every living creature, the former being congenial to it, the latter repugnant; it is through these that choice and avoidance are determined"
— Epicurus.

Humans are born helpless, needing almost total care. Fused with the mother, babies are programmed genetically to behave in ways which evoke desired responses from the mother. The mothers, in turn, are programmed to respond accordingly. Hungry babies cry. They then are given a breast or bottle and they suck vigorously. They crawl away to explore, looking back at their mother to "refuel," as Mahler puts it [op.cit 20]. They toddle across the floor into their mother's waiting arms and loving endearments. Smiles and wriggles evoke affectionate murmurs and hugs.

Humans develop by interacting with others, by learning to cause an intended result. Initially, babies please the mother with positive acts which she rewards and which give the baby a sense of achievement. Then the babies steadily expand their repertoires of transactions. They learn the behaviors which are successful and which are not and incorporate them into the beginnings of the ego and superego function.

Babies try to take control of themselves from the beginning, stopping their sucking when they want to burp or have had enough milk. The mother, in her anxiety and uncertainty, may oppose her baby's independence, pushing it to continue feeding. Thus begins the conflict with the mother for control—for autonomy—which is constant in most human relationships from birth to death.

All living organisms are programmed genetically to separate from the parent in order to survive independently and reproduce. In humans this occurs primarily between mother and child, and then with the father, siblings and other persons. Opposing the mother without estranging her is one of the more difficult tasks for the child and the mother to accept.

This conflict undergoes a crisis in the "terrible twos"—referred to by David Levy in 1954[36] as the "Opposition Syndrome" and called "Rapprochement" by Mahler[op.cit 20]. It is the time when children's frontal lobes are maturing and taking control of their behavior, L'Hermitte[37]. It is the time when children, usually on the potty or at the table, make one of life's greatest discoveries: "I don't have to do what my mother tells me. She can't make me." They discover that scolding can be tolerated, learn that their mother will sometimes ignore disobedience. In this period children will oppose anything their mothers tell them to do. "No," they say, and often do the opposite of her commands.

Through rebellion, children establish their autonomy, their identity, their ego strengths in their own minds and in the minds of their parents and the rest of the world. Usually, after one-and-a half to two years, when they have demonstrated to all concerned their ability to oppose, they no longer need to do it constantly. They have the power of choice, the ability to decide to be "bad" or "good," depending on their appraisal of the consequent pleasure or pain, the freedom to obey without jeopardizing autonomy. The conflict reaches a second critical period in adolescence when, with more independence, they anticipate leaving home. Reaching psychological adulthood they no longer defy their parents just to prove they can defy them. Perhaps the adult cuts his hair in a style he likes instead of a style his parents dislike.

The two year olds make a second discovery: they are free to try to do anything they want. They can decide what to do without reference to their mother. Her opposition becomes an element to be considered, not a determinant to the decision. They have attained freedom to do, or try to do, whatever they want.

But until they have established this option of disobedience—the power to say yes or no—children cannot choose. While still fused with their mother, they cannot distinguish what they did from what she did. Does the child eat? Or does the mother feed the child? Opposition to the mother's wishes or demands clarifies this. Now the child is in charge, now deciding, separate and independent. Decision demonstrates responsibility, a sense of authorship, of effectiveness. The child can take credit for eating. This is its achievement.

The primary function of the brain is to control behavior. A person must act, do things, in order to live and procreate "To do is to be," as Plato said. He must act to get food, warmth, companionship. A person does, or tries to do things that make him feel good. And he must be autonomous. He must do these things himself; other people cannot do them for him any more than they can breathe for him. He may do things decided or controlled by others, but at some point continued control by others weakens his mental function and ultimately leads to helplessness and insanity.

Autonomy means psychological self-government, control by the ego, the element of the brain which directs behavior. The ego is made up of consciousness, sensation, reason, the ability to choose whether to comply or oppose internal or external forces —which begins when the baby decides when or if it sucks on the maternal nipple. The ego's power is represented by will. The ego is the seat of identity, reality testing and sanity, of self-esteem and confidence. It not only controls the basic energies of hunger and sex, it has energies of its own, the energies of self-preservation.

The superego constitutes the conscience and a person's ideals of behavior. It constitutes the person's code of behavior, internalized from his parents. For control of behavior, the ego must be autonomous from the superego; a person must go through the "terrible twos" with his conscience as well as with his mother.

Conventional theory holds that ego functions, particularly a child's sense of identity, derive from identifying with others: its mother, and then father and siblings. My theory suggests that in addition to identifying, the child interacts with them and copies their behavior, particularly with peers in adolescence. Ego strengths derive from using them. This means voluntary actions controlled by the ego—doing things which have consequences in the real world. When the baby toddles successfully across the floor to its waiting mother's arms and endearments it has thereby strengthened its ego. Its achievement is twofold: motion across the floor and congratulation by its mother. Ego capacities are actually strengthened anatomically by using them. Just as muscles are strengthened by use and weakened by non use, so are ego functions. For example, the ability to remember is strengthened by use; new physical neural circuits, new neurons, develop or are lost in the cortex, amygdala and other sites in the brain. Involuntary or impulsive acts do not strengthen the ego, and may weaken it. Failure to do things results in mental disorder.

People do, or try to do, what makes them feel good. What does so is to do things which gain them rewards. They start by doing things their mothers reward; being "good." She responds with rewarding smiles, endearments, etc. These make the child feel good. The children remember the things they did which their mothers rewarded and repeat them. They so build up a superego—a repertoire of behaviors she will reward. Similarly, when they do "bad" things their mothers respond with negative rewards, scowls and punishments. These make the children feel bad, so the children learn what not to do. In this way they build up repertoires of adaptive behaviors, which they can use autonomously to get along with people. They go on to do things with other people, their family, friends, lovers. At work their methods are rewarded positively or negatively, and they modify their repertoires of behavior accordingly.

The physiological basis of reward is shown by experiments in which a lever is wired to a rat's brain reward system [39]. This is a dopaminergic projection extending from the rat's hindbrain up through the rat's midbrain, well on into the frontal lobes of the forebrain. Pressing the lever, the rat stimulates its brain reward system, causing its brain to experience "pleasure." The rat therefore presses the lever repeatedly. The rat's "ego" has found a new way to gain reward. Its autonomy is thereby strengthened.

With its mother, the child presses a psychological lever. For example, it smiles at its mother. Its mother smiles back. The lever was wired to the rat's brain. Instead of going by wire, the mother's smile goes as light-waves to the baby's eyes, and thence via optical tracts to its brain reward system. Gaining reward from smiling impels the baby to repeat the act, "presses the lever" again, e.g., smiles at its mother. Its smile is again rewarded The baby remembers smiling at the mother brings it pleasure, and so this behavior is "strengthened." The baby does other things: gurgles, wriggles. The mother responding, rewards the baby by more smiling, hugging, cries of joy, etc. She negatively rewards unadaptive behaviors; scowls, says "no." The baby feels bad, and thus learns behavior to avoid. It thus strengthens and develops adaptive behavior, strengthening autonomous ego function. The child then goes on to use its more effective behaviors with siblings, father and friends.

To develop and maintain autonomy a person must do something. Act. Cause something to happen. Especially do something that elicits a response from another person. Furthermore, he must decide for himself what he does. If he does what someone else tells him, he does not feel responsible for the consequences. Submitting to the decisions of others does not help his mental health, and may actually harm it. Of course, a person has to do what his boss tells him. But not just because the boss tells him. The person always has a choice, perhaps not a good choice, but a choice. Even to a demand, at pistol point, "Your money or your life," a person can always reply, "Well, let me think that over."

A person probably doesn't realize that these activities are what keep him sane. He does whatever makes him feel good. The concept of pleasure/reward and pain/punishment explains many areas of behavior.

This means that a person must take responsibility for what he does—take credit and risk blame—or remain forever helpless. He must be able to say, "I did it!" without refuge in blaming others. The most difficult and crucial responsibility is being honest face to face with loved ones: "Yes, I am mad at you."

"No, you can't have any more cookies."

So it is what a person does which keeps him sane, not what someone else does. For example, a patient, Mrs. J., seethed with rage at her husband. She believed he had controlled her since the day they were married. In treatment it dawned on her that the trouble was not her husband's bossiness, but her submission to his bossiness. She was realizing she could always just say "no" to his demands. She had a choice.

A person's sanity also depends on his own judgment of his behavior, not someone else's judgment. For example, a spouse may accuse him of being mean. But he judges what he is doing and arrives at his own opinion, which may differ. To some extent such autonomy can protect him from insults. Someone says, "You're a pain in the neck." In response a person can think, "Well, that's his opinion." Also a person must be able to appraise compliments. "You're wonderful!" He can ask himself, "That's nice, but why does he, or she, think so? Do I agree?" A person may get mad at someone if they dislike him, but he must ask, "Have I bored or hurt them?"

There are two main ways people confirm their opinions: by gaining agreement of another person—consensual validation—and by observing cause and effect. For example a mother says "No, you can't go out, it's raining." To the child, if she says it is raining, it must be raining. But the child may go outdoors to see for himself, holding out his hand to see if it gets wet.

But this method entails depending on one's own senses. If there is no sign of rain, if what the child perceives differs from what his mother told him, then he has to choose between trusting his own judgment or that of his mother. Questioning his mother's opinion may alarm him, may be unacceptable because he has to believe the person on whom he depends on so totally.

A patient, M., said she remembers as a small child going to the toilet and having a bowel movement. She then pulled the chain and watched the movement go down the drain. This was a new achievement for her. She rushed to her nurse and proudly reported what she had done. The nurse, skeptical, went and looked in the toilet and seeing no bowel movement, disbelieved her story. '"But I saw it go down the drain," cried M. M.'s mother was called to adjudicate. The mother sided with the nurse and M. was given an enema. M. said she never forgot that event. Poor M. Who was she to believe ? Her own eyes and ears? Or the chief authorities in her world?

Methods for validating cognitive processes are used constantly throughout a lifetime. The extent that conviction relies on agreement from other people has profound influence on self-confidence and relationships. The essence of autonomy is use of one's own perceptions to test reality.

Autonomy might be thought to be the same as "self-assertion." However deciding for himself what he will do or think is not the same pushing or intruding on others. Assertive demands may be simply the expression of a need. The cry of a dependent infant is certainly assertive and impels others to satisfy it. On the other hand, when an autonomous adult is assertive, he takes into account the effect on others, a deliberate action to solve a problem or reach a goal.

Since man is a social animal, most of the acts which maintain a person's autonomy and mental health are interactions with other people. They strengthen, defend and maintain ego strength and control. They bring feelings of pleasure, confidence, success, achievement; feelings of value, of importance, sexual success, of being loved; a sense of social acceptance, of belonging to a group, of respect from family members and peers.

To interact means to act upon one another. Each person causes an effect in the other. Interaction means reciprocal action. When a person smiles at someone, the recipient of his smile does something to him in response, not necessarily a returning smile, but some action which in turn affects the person who smiled. One may not ordinarily think of smiling or scowling as doing something to another person. But a smile, or a scowl, or a tear, affects a recipient. A person is not helpless, he has power to make the other person respond in some way, even if not always the way he wants.

Being active in nonsocial activities also, to a limited extent, enables a person to stay sane. For example doing physics, or gardening, or learning a language can help his mental health considerably. But things do not actively respond to what a person does. He can not make a thing act. People react and a person has power to make them do so. This is why social interaction is necessary for sanity.

A strong ego is one which has a repertoire of behaviors to attract other people. This includes the entire vast array of all human interaction—greeting someone, making eye-contact, touching, talking, listening, etc. Most such interactions are transactions or intended transactions: a smile to beget a smile, a complaint to beget sympathy, a scowl to beget a retreat. Most are intended, at the least, to get attention, a little understood, but powerful phenomena. It brings people to life, energizes them as though plugged into an electric socket.

Such social interaction is complex and involves an immense number of elements. Scientists can explain the physical world as the interaction of charged particles, electrons, protons, quarks, etc. The elements of human communication have been too vast and intricate for the same kind of analysis. Birdwhistle[40] analyzed films of two individuals conversing and identified over a thousand transactions per minute. This number seems implausible when first considered. But it includes the subtle, subliminal interactions involving body language, facial expression, tones of voice, pauses between spoken words, eye language—all the elements of affective as well as cognitive communication.

A friendly look involves the expressions of the face, the position of the eyebrows, the duration of the eye contact, the person's posture. A friendly tone of voice has a range of wave lengths. The configuration of the eyebrows is different in a hostile look; they slant downward from the outside to the inside of the face. Charles Darwin[41] described the facial expressions in basic affects such as anger, fear, and mirth. The very high level of sensitivity in human communication upon which mental health depends is illustrated by the observation that within a day, if a newborn has been in continuous contact with the mother, within hours it can recognize her voice and differentiate it from other women's voices. Similarly a mother can distinguish the sound of her infant's cry among other infants. The wave lengths denoting degree of warmth of a mother's voice are being related to subsequent behavior of daughters in adulthood—such as the number of children they choose to bear[42].

The complexity of interaction helps explain the difficulties of communication between people, and the frequency of miscommunications and misunderstandings. Billions of cells in the brain's biologic computer are required to perceive and respond and interact socially. Hearing begins with a physical experience —sound waves hitting the ear drum, for example. Despite this mysterious, almost infinitely complicated conjunction of the physical and emotional, people do manage to interact, do develop social skills, do "win friends and influence people."

A sense of responsibility is what develops the ego, delivering a feeling of effectiveness, of identity. I am he—or she—who does things, who eats, who walks. I am a person who raises a family, who works and produces results. The minuscule, momentary actions in a person's daily intimate life also serve in this respect —scratching one's nose, brushing one's teeth, choosing a white shirt instead of blue, saying "hello" to someone. However, other actions may weaken the ego. If people submit to the decisions of another person, they do not feel responsible for the consequences. The person who makes the decision, either one's self, or the other person, is responsible. Also, if emotions take control, if people lose their temper or run away in panic, they do not accept responsibility—"I couldn't help it!"

Conventional psychoanalytic theory holds that unconscious forces frequently influence people's behaviors, and on occasion determine actions. Man has had three blows to his pride: first Copernicus showed that Man is not the center of the universe. Then Darwin showed that He descended from monkeys. Then Freud said that Man is not even master in his own being, but is controlled by unconscious forces in his nature. However, I suggest that in autonomous persons the unconscious does not control behavior. As Freud himself said, "Where Id was, Ego shall be," which means where passions were, reason will be. The ego is primarily conscious. Its forces of reason and will are definitively powerful and in control. Action and interaction are crucial to maintaining autonomy, even when people are propelled by motives they do not fully comprehend, do not admit to themselves—vanity, greed, lust, fear, rage, selfishness, etc. Nevertheless, minute by minute in daily life, they do make conscious decisions. Whether their reasons are right or wrong, they have authored an action, an effect, and feel responsible for the consequences, feel pride or guilt or blame.

Ego strengths and ego autonomy are not the same. People may have powerful ego capacities for reasoning, a strong will, great knowledge, great self confidence, even arrogance, yet, like a child, not be good at taking care of themselves. They may depend heavily on someone else for this, even letting another decide what clothes to wear or how to spend their money. Conversely, relatively simple people, uneducated, modest, may run their own lives quite adequately. The sanity of the brilliant, arrogant, but dependent person may be less stable than that of a meek but adult neighbor.

In any relationship a person intuitively tests the autonomy of the other and adjusts accordingly. For example, he tests whether the other compulsively needs to be always right. Or they can listen to what he says with an open mind. Such freedom is sought by everybody. He hates being controlled, told what to think and do. He hates constantly giving in. He may not recognize the reason he reacts so strongly. His mental health is involved. He is defending his sanity.

Conscience, the judgmental self, is a mother's rules internalized, the imprint of her commands and interdictions. Its decrees are shaped originally by the need to please the mother and get rewards. "Right" means parental approval, "wrong" means disapproval punishable by "castration," abandonment, or whatever. Though people do not ordinarily connect right and wrong with parental approval; in their minds, being wrong is being wrong, and to question why is unthinkable.

A person must go through the terrible twos, first with his mother, then with his conscience. An adolescent must "sow his wild oats," do bad things, smoke, get drunk, talk back, hurt somebody's feelings, perhaps even cheat and steal, kiss girls, masturbate, do anything "bad" to evaluate his conscience's rules.

He also must do "good" things, be considerate of others, be honest, etc. He tests the rules on himself, sees whether they work for him in his life, sees the consequences of complying with or opposing them. He shifts from trusting authority to trusting his observation of cause and effect.

Failure to do so results in mental disorder. Automatically submitting to "the rules" and constantly letting the dictates of conscience override his own judgment is equivalent to depending endlessly on his external mother or other persons to make decisions for him. When submitting to his conscience he is not responsible for his actions. Causality is not involved, "I didn't do anything, I was just doing my duty," which is similar to saying "don't blame me, she made me do it."

An adult has become autonomous from his mother and from his mother's rules and has developed his own patterns of behavior to gain reward. He can choose whether to comply or oppose his conscience, just as he can choose whether to comply with or oppose his mother. He then can can feel responsible for his actions.

An adult can prevent his feelings from controlling him. To do so he must realize he may be angry without knowing it, or frightened, or unaware that he is making sexual advances. He, like everyone, is profoundly influenced by motives and beliefs buried in his unconscious. For example, he may hold "choice" in abortion as a cause to live or die for—and be quite unaware that his passion comes from experience with his mother, who never allowed him to choose anything. Similarly, a person's passionate insistence on privacy may come from his lack of it as a child. A person's basic expectations of getting rewards from others may come from his success—or failure—as a child trying to please his mother. Knowing that all people are full of unconscious prejudices, rationalizations and biases may enable a person to tolerate irrationalities in others—and in himself.

So sanity includes autonomy not only from demands of other people and from "shoulds," but also from compelling emotions: temper, fear, lust, greed. A person cannot control whether he has these feelings, only what he does about them.

In summary, my theory is based on the concept of autonomous action and interaction. Man is what he does. He survives by doing things to obtain what he needs from his environment: food, shelter, and social interplay.

CHAPTER THREE

LESLIE

Clinical Examples

The following three chapters present verbatim excerpts from the cases of three patients. These have been selected to illustrate the role of autonomy in mental disorder: 1) The lack of autonomy and resultant helplessness, 2) how this was caused in childhood from interacting with parents, and 3) how, in the course of treatment, the patients interacting with their physician gained autonomy and then lived normal lives.

The means used by their physician in this interaction will be elaborated on in Chapter 7. Aspects of the patient's disorders other than those of autonomy have not been focused upon. This approach to the patient's disorders differs from current theory, chiefly by its focus on decision making and behavior as contrasted with motives and feelings.

Leslie's self-mutilation was a declaration, to show her external and internalized parents that she had a mind and emotions of her own, especially rage. The turning point of Professor Marsh's treatment was the day he disobeyed his mother. The case of Elinor was all about opposition, her inability to go against the wishes of her family.

The actual statements and actions of the patients and the physician are presented in bold type. The thoughts of the physician are in regular type.

The Self Cutter, the Strangler

A 23-year-old female law-student named Leslie is brought to the hospital struggling in the arms of her father. She has knocked on the door of her parents' bedroom and thrust in their faces a deep, bleeding cut, three inches long, deliberately done on her forearm with a razor blade.

Why did she cut herself? And why show her parents? Was she mad at them? Did she expect them to help her? At a later time she said cutting herself was the only way she could think of to get their attention .

In the hospital she is kept constantly in full physical restraints, including arms, legs and body. Otherwise, she will assault anyone in sight, bang her head against the wall, or attempt again to cut herself.

Why assault people? Was she seeking autonomy?

On an occasion after attempting to strangle a nurse, Leslie is asked why she did it. She says, "I didn't do it. Emma did it." Emma, a male in her imagination, is the name she sometimes calls herself. Asked why Emma did it, she says, "Because the Black Lord told him to."

Here was a double denial of responsibility. In her mind Leslie had not assaulted the nurse. Emma had. Emma merely did what the "Black Lord" commanded. Blaming Emma, Leslie had psychologically by-passed the circuits of her ego. Since assaulting a nurse was unacceptable to her, she had repressed her ego involvement.

One day, while struggling in full restraints, she said, "It feels so good to fight as hard as I can and yet know I can't hurt myself or anybody else." Unable to control her own movements she welcomed external control.

The first day in the hospital I talk with her father. He tells

me, "The key to the problem is the fact that her mother contracted phlebitis at Leslie's birth. She had wanted a boy, not a girl, and blamed Leslie for her phlebitis. She has never been able to take care of Leslie and there has always been hostility between them."

In Leslie's experience the mother/child interaction had been deficient. When she acted to evoke nurturance, her mother failed to reward her—which made Leslie angry at her mother—who therefore gave even less care. The vicious cycle sabotaged development of adequate social function.

In that first session her father says, "Leslie had tantrums over brushing her teeth at age six."

Tantrums of this type are usually paradigmatic of autonomy conflict between mother and child. The mother attempts to force the child to brush her teeth and over-does it, threatening the child's autonomy, sparking rebellion. This in turn impels the mother, already angry at the child, to enforce the tooth-brushing even more vigorously, triggering a tantrum, a desperate struggle to maintain autonomy.

Her father said that Leslie believes everybody in her class hated her: "She never had any friends. She never opened up to anyone."

Leslie was incapable of intimacy, could not make friends since she had no repertoire of ways to attract others.

At the end this visit I ask her father if he planned to visit Leslie the next day.

I thought that he would want to see and comfort her after she had such a terrifying day, cutting her arm, being locked up in a mental hospital. She might need, desperately, to see him.

"Oh no," he says. He has to "officiate" the next day and is unable to visit her.

By bringing his daughter to the hospital, he had met her need to be taken care of and controlled. But he was now too busy with his important affairs to recognize and respond to his daughter's further need to be comforted and loved by him. This suggested a pattern of basic failure to meet her needs which could have left Leslie helpless. It was noteworthy, too, that he blamed Leslie's difficulties on his wife's phlebitis, thus denying any responsibility on his part. This suggested no awareness of his wife's intimate internal struggles. I noted that he—not her mother—had brought Leslie to the hospital and talked to me. Why? Was her mother not strong enough? Or uncaring? Her failure could further contribute to Leslie's sense of helplessness.

The next day in her session with me, Leslie immediately asks, "Did my father tell you about their not bringing me up?"

Why did Leslie ask me this? She believes they did not bring her up, but is very unsure of her judgment. If her father told me so I might believe it—which would validate her judgment. There are two main ways people confirm their opinions: by gaining agreement of another person—consensual validation—and by observing cause and effect. For example, a mother says, "No, you can't go out, it's raining." To the child, if she says it is raining, it must be raining. But the child may go outdoors to see for himself, holding out his hand to see if it gets wet.

But this method entails depending on one's own senses. If there is no sign of rain, if what the child perceives differs from what his mother told him, then he has to choose between trusting his own judgment or that of his mother. Questioning his mother's opinion may alarm him, may be unacceptable because he has to believe the person on whom he depends so totally.

Methods for validating cognitive processes are used constantly throughout a lifetime. The extent that conviction relies on agreement from other people has profound influence on self-confidence and relationships. The essence of autonomy is the use of one's own perceptions to test reality.

Leslie asked me this question to seek my agreement. If I agreed, then her opinion was validated. She might then believe she was correct.

I answered her question. "Yes," I replied, "he did tell me."

I thus rewarded her autonomous act of asking me a question. This established the pattern of my treatment. She could learn she was not helpless, rather she had the power to elicit responses from me.

Leslie says her father is a person who can't sit still. He must always be on the go, and he never listens.

Coupled with being too busy, too absorbed in his own affairs, too self-centered to visit his daughter, this implied to Leslie that what she said or wanted was not worth considering. If her own father would not listen to her, how could she expect any one else to listen? Feeling that she was never listened to contributed to her inability "to open up" and be capable of intimate relationships.

Leslie also says that her father wants to make decisions for her, about law school, or any career. That is all he cares about. She is the fifth generation bearing her father's name, and though "merely a girl," she must carry on the family tradition of success.

Her father's expectations for career performance, denying her the right to make choices, deprecated her gender and had no reference to her interests or ability. This undermined her self-confidence, and suggested that he regarded her as simply a vehicle for continued family achievement. If she failed in this, she was of little value to him.

Leslie says her main fear is that when she tells me things, I will answer that there's nothing the matter with her, that she'll grow out of it—which her father had been telling her for years.

Our relationship, the father-transference, had begun. Leslie had expected me to behave like her own father, who neither listened to nor validated what she might say. She had little confidence that anything she thought was true. Could she convince me? The validity of her thoughts was at stake. If I, her doctor, dismissed her thinking, then what hope had she?

She says, "It's so amazing that you listen to me. It's the best thing that has happened in my life."

"Amazing" because no one has listened to her before. It is "best" because listening validated her thinking. I rewarded the act of talking to me, made her less helpless; afforded her some power to affect me. My "listening" was not passive, but active, responding to her speech with all the complex elements of social interaction, including facial expressions, tones of voice, as well as replying to her questions and comments.

She goes on to tell me that her father claims that he and her mother have the perfect marriage. She thinks her mother, in fact, has always been miserable. Her mother once told Leslie that she would like to press the "bomb button"—an atomic bomb that would blow up her husband and the world.

How could she trust a mother who wanted to blow up the whole family, Leslie concluded. Why was her mother so explosively angry? Did Leslie believe she, herself was to blame? Merely because she was alive and needing nurturance from her mother? Merely because she was not the boy her mother and father wanted?

In addition, Leslie was expressing an opinion which strongly disagreed with one of her father's major convictions. The dichotomy between her judgment and her father's must have made her doubt her own vision of the marriage, doubt her own perceptions.

Both parents would disagree violently with what she told me about their marriage. What was she to believe? Would I side with her or her parents? To become sane, able to run her life, Leslie would have to gain confidence in the correctness of her own thinking and decisions. **I sided with her opinions regularly as a pattern of my treatment, differing with her only when her opinions seemed clearly mistaken.**

Leslie tells me she can't stand any physical contact or expression of affection.

This represented major pathology. Affection endangered Leslie's identity, her sense of "I," without which a person no longer exists. Since Leslie had little autonomy, her identity was extremely fragile, vulnerable to engulfment by other persons. So affection was a setup for the domination which imperiled her very existence. Although desperately lonely, any friendly approach frightened her.

Leslie says, "I don't know what to do when I get angry; I have two choices: injure myself, or bash the other person." She adds in an urgent voice, "Don't ever ask me what you should do at such times. I was so grateful when you just left and locked the door the other day."

Usually, during our sessions Leslie could control her behavior. But that time she attacked me physically, I escaped from her room and locked the door. I understood that I must not ask for impossible decisions and control. Autonomy includes the ability to manage one's temper, and in this respect Leslie was nearly helpless. So her violence had to be controlled by external means, just as a mother must sometimes control her child.

She tells me that at age four she pushed a woman, who fell backward down a flight of stairs and knocked out two front teeth. The woman was the daughter of her nurse, who blamed Leslie for the accident and punished her by repeatedly and painfully taking off a bandage which Leslie had on her knee.

Experiences of this kind led her to fear the harm that her anger might cause, so she directed it inward rather than outward. But following this session with me, Leslie became actively assaultive and was placed in an intensive-care unit. There she struggled violently for an hour against two attendants who were preventing her from banging her head on the wall.

During the first year, Leslie was immobilized with physical restraints. When staff was available, I had her controlled manually by nurses or attendants. She seemed able to tolerate, even welcome, human touch when used in this way. Perhaps that did not endanger her identity. Also, nurses were usually able to restrain her in a friendly way, so her anger served to bring her closer to people.

Discussing the day she was restrained after attacking me, Leslie says she could have kept fighting all day and all night. She says she often has the impulse to bang her head when I leave at the end of my visits.

The reasons for this are not clear. She was frustrated and angry with me for leaving her at the end of my visits. The visits lasted almost an hour, but she almost always seemed to want me to stay longer. The day she recalled knocking out the teeth of her nurse's daughter, her anger was no doubt increased at the memory.

Leslie says, "I shred people in my mind. I take off their ears, then pull off their skin, then I pull out their brains. I've

done this for years." She adds, "I always dream the same dream: I am about to be executed for some crime."

Leslie was now opening up to me. "Shredding" was undoubtedly one of her crimes. Her parents would have responded with horror, told her she should not have such feelings, thereby increasing her guilt. **In contrast, I sought to understand the cause of her anger.** Doing so implied there was a cause, which made her feel less guilty. **At the same time I protected myself and protected her from her anger with physical and pharmacological restraints.** In this way she could develop intimacy with me.

Leslie tells me that her mother has over a hundred doll houses on the third floor of their house. These are exquisitely furnished and kept in perfect order and cleanliness. But there are no dolls in them. In addition, Leslie tells me a dream in which she was standing on an oriental rug and bleeding. Scolding her furiously, her mother was not concerned about her, only that she was soiling the rug with her blood. She says this is typical of her mother.

The chief point was the indifference to her welfare. It took blood to catch her mother's attention. Clearly blood had an important meaning to her. The dream was not clear about the source of the blood, whether from a cut or whether she was menstruating and therefore Oedipal rivalry might be an issue.

In the hospital Leslie refuses to urinate for prolonged periods, even though on examination her bladder is over-full, and she is in obvious distress. She walks around the hospital with an in-dwelling catheter and plastic urinal strapped to her leg. She has similar difficulty defecating, and would go for long periods without a bowel movement, even though clearly in distress. She says she knows this trouble comes from the cruel

way her parents handled her during toilet training. She says she can't talk about it. It's just too upsetting.

She is given enemas, but even so, she sometimes waits so long that her feces became impacted and have to be extracted manually, a painful and messy process, both for her and the nurses who do it. In fact the nurses, though concerned, are rebellious.

It was never clear whether Leslie did not urinate and defecate because she could not or because she would not. Clearly, she took satisfaction from the nurse's concern—and consternation. Their reaction seemed to be an element of her therapy. Leslie was reliving the experience in bowel training she had had with her mother who was more concerned with getting these functions performed than with Leslie's autonomy.

The same pattern occurs in her feeding. **She refuses to eat, so she is fed. She resists this, turning her head away or spitting out the food placed in her mouth. So she is fed by a tube put down through her nose. Even here she has to be kept in restraints, otherwise she will pull out the tube—oppositional behavior with a vengeance.**

Leslie's self-injury was a way to seek nurturance, while preserving her autonomy and expressing her fury at her mother. **When nurses would come running and struggled with her, they did not tell her to stop banging her head and to control herself. They accepted her struggle. When she refused to eat, her physician did not reason with her. The nurses inserted a tube down her throat and poured in the food. In both cases the physical intervention was done to her.**

This is analogous to a parent dealing with a child who refuses to go to bed. The parent urges the child to go, orders it to go, but after a certain point gives up and simply carries the child to bed. In this way the child has not done it, the parent has. The child's autonomy has been preserved.

During the course of treatment, Leslie's pattern of maintaining her autonomy by opposition, assaultiveness and self-destructiveness was gradually abandoned as she found more effective ways to interact, based on our interaction. She began eating and performing her bodily functions on her own. Presumably she had proved her autonomy and could act because she wanted to, not because she was obedient.

Early in her stay, while she is struggling with attendants, I hear her say "my precious" several times in a low voice. When she has quieted down, I ask her about this. Over the ensuing months she introduces me to "The Kingdom," based on J.R.R. Tolkein's novel: *The Lords of the Ring.*

The Kingdom was ruled by a White Lord, representing good, although a fierce kind of good, and by a Black Lord, representing evil, rage, revenge, selfishness. His existence was so secret, that months passed before Leslie told me about him. Lesser Lords played roles. There was a kindly, somewhat ineffective Lord, who represented Leslie's family doctor.

The Black Lord lived in Mordor from whence he fought the White Lord. His power was contained in a magic ring. A "little person" named Frodo had gained possession of the magic ring, which he called "My Precious," and he was trying to take it to a volcanic cauldron which would destroy it. Leslie saw herself as Frodo, poor weak Frodo. Struggling with the attendants in the hospital, the minions of the Black Lord, she was the ring bearer.

Leslie talks to me extensively about her adventures in The Kingdom: how she escaped capture by the agents of the Black Lord, how she suffered the punishment imposed on her by the White Lord for various transgressions and shortcomings—an

echo of her super-ego. She seems to gain deep satisfaction from my interest in these accounts.

Telling me about "The Kingdom," Leslie discovered that she could safely interact with me. I did not behave toward her like the Lords. I did not admonish her or rage at her. I was not as condemning of the Black Lord as she expected me to be. I was simply interested in why he was so angry. She saw, too, that I dared to question The White Lord, and even disagreed with him at times when his pronouncements seemed unduly harsh. Learning to interact with me, she gradually learned to interact with other people. Changing Leslie's code of behavior, her definitions of right and wrong—the legacy of her mother and father—was very difficult. But when she projected her code onto her physician during interaction, she began to perceive, consciously and unconsciously, that there was a difference, and she could begin to adopt elements of his code.

With years of continued treatment she became able to control herself and take responsibility for what she did. She no longer blamed Emma and The Lords. She learned how to talk to people, to function autonomously. She no longer was weird looking, no longer self-destructive. She was discharged from the hospital, and with further continued treatment as an out-patient, she ceased to be shy, stopped making others uncomfortable, ended her helplessness, her inability to defend herself. She graduated from medical school, and became a physician. Some years later she writes, "I am busy and happy and look forward to seeing some private patients in the not too distant future."

CHAPTER FOUR

THE UPSIDE DOWN PROFESSOR

Professor Marsh, an eminent theoretical physicist, appeared at the office of the president of his University and demanded to see him immediately. The professor was sweating and excited. He demanded that the president immediately telephone the White House and tell the President to order the National Science Foundation to set up a plan for teaching physics to high school students. He was taken to the infirmary, where he told the doctor that he had been communicating by brain waves with a woman, Judith, and she had agreed to marry him. He was referred to me for treatment.

The professor was clearly out of his mind. Why did he have such grandiose ideas and demands? Why did he have to appeal to such high authority? He must be feeling helpless. And why did he have to invoke "brain waves," supernatural means, to talk with a girl friend? He must fear she would refuse to talk to him face to face. His grandiosity made him feel less helpless, provided him with an illusion of power.

Over the telephone the professor agrees to come to my hospital, but says he does not want his parents to accompany him. "I want to feel independent," he explains.

This statement suggested that the professor had an autonomy conflict with his parents: they opposed his desire for independence. The fact that he told me this almost as a condition for coming to the hospital suggested that independence was very important to him—and that he was overly dependent on his parents, a "mama's boy" who was struggling to break free.

Also, Professor Marsh's eager willingness to check into the hospital suggested that he felt helpless and was also very trusting, perhaps overly so. He did not know me personally, although I had been recommended by his university.

Professor Marsh is a smallish, somewhat plump man wearing a red necktie. He has large blue eyes, a quiet intense voice. He asks me whether my accent is English. I say no, "I got it in Cambridge, Massachusetts, and I was born in New York City."

This response rewarded Professor Marsh. I had answered and added an elaboration. He had found that asking a question was an effective way of interacting with me.

He tells me that his accent was acquired in Natick, Massachusetts, he had been born in Brooklyn, New York, then went to Ithaca, and finally moved to Natick and attended MIT. Having established a degree of personal relationship with me, he goes on to say that he has been upset. "I did some peculiar things," he said, "but my life has been quieting down in the last few days." He talks of his intensity when writing his memorandum for the University President, seventy-five pages in four days detailing his plan for teaching physics in the nation's high schools.

Why was writing the report so urgent?

Next he talks about his personal life, saying that he wanted to marry a certain girl if she would have him. "I have decided to give up Physics," he says. "I want to keep my professorship, but ask for extended leave, go to England, perhaps Washington. Also turn my interest to other subjects that have interested me, mathematics, history. For example I want to finish some books by Kennan, Churchill's history of World War Two.

I comment, "Turn toward people."

"Yes," he says. "In physics I find I can talk to a few physicists, but not to many other people. You keep people away. Some people one can talk to. I find I can talk to you."

My comment "Turn toward people" was a response to his loneliness, his social helplessness, his desperate attempts to interact. He was like Leslie, keeping people away, identifying intimacy with danger, the threat of domination and loss of identity. Yet his identity depended on interacting with people

He tells me that the report he gave to the President of his University was upsetting because . . . he stops and asks, "Is it all right for me to talk freely?" I tell him that what he says is confidential. He tells me the physics department used to be the best in the country, but has been slipping and they need to make three appointments. In the report he cited the limitations of certain members of the physics department. Some were friends and he feels guilty.

These comments revealed the immediate cause of Professor Marsh's breakdown: failure at work due to doubts about his judgment. It made clear why writing to the president was so urgent. As department chairman, he had to make decisions which evoked resentment and challenges from colleagues. If they thought he was wrong, how could he oppose them? Perhaps he should not be chairman of the department. It was therefore urgent to seek support from higher authority.

Asking if it was "all right to talk freely" suggested that he is placing trust in me as his physician, and believes that I will side with him rather than with his bitter colleagues.

Continuing, the Professor says his thinking is clearing up because he is changing certain values—turning more toward people rather than physicists. If the girl he wants to marry

turns him down, he will be disappointed, but not dismayed. He will seek another girl. I ask why he has delayed marriage until now. He replies, "Interest in physics, utter engrossment in it."

His use of the phrase "turning toward people" echoes my previous comment and indicates extreme suggestibility, a willingness to let me control his thinking. His comment that his interest in physics kept him away from "love" suggests a pattern only too common in scientists: an inability to form intimate relationships causes them to substitute work for satisfaction, particularly scientific work which involves minimal social competence.

Professor Marsh tells me that he did not marry earlier because the kind of girl he liked would not want to marry a person like him, would not appreciate physics and would not be satisfied with the small income of a young scientist.

So Professor Marsh believed that without money or prestige, he had little to offer women. His personal qualities, appearance, charm, intelligence, character, counted for little. He knew no way to please women.

In psychosis, psychic structure has broken down, causing an inability to perceive reality. Because his power to decide and act had been impaired, Professor Marsh feared that any action would be inept and bound to fail. If he tried to go somewhere, he would get lost. If he tried to talk, he would be misunderstood, evoke hostility, or, worst of all, be ignored. Any interaction would end in disaster, in being hurt or humiliated. My goal in treating him must be to reward his attempts to interact

He tells me that his parents always thought he was wrong to be in academic life. His father is a businessman, a vice-president of a Life Insurance Company. That is why Professor Marsh did not want his parents to come with him to the hospital.

I ask, "They tend to confuse you? Make you feel that even now you have chosen the wrong career?"

He answers, "Yes."

Here the etiology emerged, the cause of his helplessness. His parents told him that his judgment was faulty, that his choice of career was a mistake, even though he was a world class physicist at a top university. They continued to undermine his confidence and were dangerous to his sanity.

Though Professor Marsh needed their love, he was not capable of a love that involved interaction between two persons. A sense of autonomy and responsibility are essential elements in attachment between people. Then the love they get maintains their sense of self.

Shall he begin at the beginning? Professor Marsh tells me that he majored in electrical engineering at M.I.T. Then he served in the army in World War II, and at the end of that time was "tired of being told what to do, of being pushed around. I decided to do what I wanted to do for a change." He continues, "I returned to M.I.T. In engineering they told me I had to do a lot of lab work. Well, I wasn't about to do that. In theoretical physics I could do what I wanted. It is a pretty subject, and also certain—not like history where one can just have an opinion. In physics the answers are "right."

His striking words were "tired of being told what to do, of being pushed around." This, I believed, was the essence of the Professor's pathology. Feeling in constant danger of losing his identity, he struggled desperately to resist external control. I suspected this was the story of his life.

Very likely Professor Marsh's superb ability to think was developed as a means of achieving autonomy, of proving to himself that indeed he was able to think despite his mother's dismissal of his opinions. He chose theoretical physics because there is always a definite answer to a problem. But for Professor Marsh, that was the catch. In the end, his own opinion did not matter. The answer was already there to be discovered, proven correct. Being a distinguished physicist was ultimately not enough for him, did not prove that he was indeed able to decide daily things for himself.

His next statement, "I decided to do what I wanted, for a change," confirmed that he had been doing only what others wanted. Because he had little confidence in his ability to defend his opinion against disagreement, Professor Marsh was attracted by science where answers are provably "right."

In this first interview Professor Marsh had somewhat regained control of himself. His behavior toward me was socially appropriate though unduly dependent and confiding. There were no reference to "brain waves," or other signs of gross cognitive defects. But his underlying psychosis was evident. He had lost his ability to test reality and was unable to take care of himself.

My diagnose was Schizophrenic Reaction, Undifferentiated, in partial remission. Basic elements in the dynamics of his psychosis were suggested.

Treatment will involve his gaining control of his thoughts and behavior, particularly the ability to attract other people and to oppose control by other people.

The course of his treatment will be illustrated in the following excerpts of his sessions with me over the following 2 years.

The next day he is very worried because he had not phoned his parents, despite promising them. He says his relations with his parents are critical. He must avoid seeing them. He wants me to avoid them also.

Professor Marsh was dramatizing the conflict between autonomy and love, the "double-bind" described by Jackson. His parents' anger was terrifying, but obeying them jeopardized his sanity. Moreover, he did not want me to see them either. He worried that they would control my thinking about him, my decisions. I would become their ally, not his. He was talking here about his social isolation. He was now extending his fear—control by his parents—to control by people in general.

Professor Marsh explains, "My mother is very intelligent, but she has never had enough contact with other intelligent people. So she is very opinionated. She feels no need to justify her opinions." She is treating him as though he is a child, telling him when to go to bed, when to wear an overcoat."

For the first time he specified his mother alone as the controller, not both his parents. The danger to sanity comes from submission, not from the bossiness of another person. The professor did not have to behave like a child. Theoretically, he had the option to oppose his mother and decide for himself what he did.

During our next session, the Professor says, "I've been studying this place, the lines of authority. I'm with people I can push around . . . I cannot dominate you . . . I'd like to leave tomorrow because of the discomfort on the floor . . . the size of the cups is a sign that I should take a smaller amount of medicine. I would like to move to a lower floor where there is more freedom." He appeared confused, overly tense, helpless.

Professor Marsh was moved to a locked floor for more disturbed patients.

A few days later he says he likes his new floor. much better . . . more room to scheme . . . less social pressure. He is no longer so concerned about dominating people . . . says he is communicating with Judith via brain waves . . . feels like she is

in this country [Judith is British and lives in England]. . . . He thinks I am very subtle in my arrangements, for having Doctor X placed as a patient on the ward.

Patient's father visits patient. Afterwards his father tells me his son had a "fierce desire for independence after leaving the army." He also says his son would do "silly things," such as fly to the west coast and back in one day to attend a scientific meeting (which in fact is not infrequent among academics).

There was now a diagnostic puzzle: how could Professor Marsh's autonomy have been so severely impaired by his parents, while at the same time his cognitive capacities were developed to the degree that he was a world level theoretical physicist? His inability to talk to his parents led him to think things through on his own, thereby to reassure himself of the validity of his own thinking.

Children ordinarily validate their thinking by gaining their mothers' agreement. When that is not forthcoming, they may confirm it other ways: by logic, by observing the consequences, by a positive reaction in the world of physics. His ability to talk to his father gave the Professor Marsh some validation of his cognitive capacities. Doubtless, this led him to keep trying to think for himself, rather than give up altogether.

A colleague also visits. Professor Marsh tells me he thinks the colleague was reassured about him, by the visit, and will reassure other members of the physics department

Professor Marsh is clearly worried about the effect of his breakdown on his colleagues. They in turn are indeed very worried about him. These colleagues—also world level scientists—are very concerned about him, their chairman. Throughout his stay in the hospital they visit and write to him and play no small part in his recovery.

The next day he says he likes to walk around without his shoes . . . says he does this a lot at home. . . . feels he's seeing things in better perspective . . . is full of zest and desire to do things, full of schemes. He's decided he would like to be chairman of the department, but not teach any courses so he will have time for other activities. . . . still feels too immersed in physics and wants to go to art galleries, sit in on some history courses.

The next day he says he feels fine . . . things seem to be steadily clearer . . . about himself, me, his situation. He is afraid of a tendency to dominate people, but says "I don't like to think about it." He continues, "My mother has a tendency to dominate me. She's the only person I'm close to that I'm unable to talk to. You can't reason with her. I would never tell her about Judith (the woman he is considering to marry)." My mother has a tendency to treat me as a child; about such things as time of going to bed, wearing rubbers and so on."

The army had considerable influence on him.. first time he felt independent..lived at home going to college. I say, his mother is the kind of person who finds it difficult to relinquish her children. Exactly, replies Professor Marsh

He's eager to get on with his plans, but says, "I didn't want to see my mother because she makes me feel weak, as though I can be easily pushed around . . . and could become dependent." But now he thinks he can cope with her. He feels stronger, more able to take care of himself. He does not want to be chairman of the physics department next year, and not even teach classes. He wants time to travel.

Professor Marsh is improving rapidly. Not only is he beginning to understand his mother's power to make him feel weak-willed, helpless, but feeling "stronger" meant that somehow he could manage to do what he—not his mother—decided.

Day 13

Says he has difficulty admitting he's mentally ill. . . . As he improves he sees how far off he was on many things

Nurses report he stares in a way which upsets his roommate, but otherwise his behavior is normal.

Day 16

Says he would like to get back to his University as soon as possible. [He looks brighter and stronger] . . . says he had a wonderful visit with his father...eager to return to his University. During the next ten days he kept repeating an urgent desire to return to his University

Professor Marsh had reconstituted considerably. Although he was far from ready to resume his duties, I decided to agree to a visit home in order to reward his improvement, and more important, enable him to discover for himself that he was still unwell and in need of further treatment. He then could assume responsibility for being in the hospital.

Day 27

Allowed to leave hospital with friends to visit over the weekend. For a day he seemed to them to be normal. The next morning seemed confused, particularly regarding time. The next day he seemed normal until evening. He suddenly had a tantrum, threw himself on the floor in front of guests, and talked of wanting to reform the world. He was returned to the hospital.

During the next few days, he tells me that he is confused about which is east and which is west. He says he has been thinking about Judith and about America. So excited. That's why he did those silly things at his friends. They probably phoned me. "My eyes click. . . . I think I tend to stare too much at people. I need more people to talk to, I need to talk to you

more. . . . I have electrical sensations. . . . I'm letting you dominate me. . . . I have a feeling that a good deal is going on that I'm not being told about." And it was at this time he said," I AM UPSIDE DOWN." He also said, "I heard someone talk about sex therapy and that I would never agree to this." At a later time he asked, in an excited voice, and sweating heavily, "When does sex therapy begin?" . . . He said, "I feel I have strings coming out of my face."... He said, "I would like to see my parents, also Margie K " a girl I was very close to for seven to eight years. She turned me down. She required I turn Catholic and I declined to. Thereby losing a woman's love because he did not submit to her demands **As he said this he copied my posture, crossing his legs, folding his hands in his lap. Asked why he did this he said, "Because of sex therapy."**

It is clear from the above his psychosis had returned. That he was "upside down" is cited here merely to indicate the degree of his disorientation. He repeated this statement intermittently during the next few weeks, but its dynamics did not become clear and it is not cited as a key feature of his illness in this respect. His reference to sex therapy is of course interesting and suggests a dynamic role for sexuality in his illness. The role of sexuality in Professor M.'s psychosis never did become clear, but will be discussed further subsequently. Its significance here is perhaps suggested by his statement that he would never agree to it, which refers to his autonomy and my ability to "dominate" him. Perhaps his copying my posture meant he was under my domination so could engage in sex without responsibility for doing so.

Day 36

Nurses report patient dribbling food in a way which disturbed other patients. Says he feels calmer when I visit him . . .

his eyes flicker . . . he thinks he's calming down very quickly . . . Felicia said she'd come visit him again next Sunday

Here are excerpts of sessions over the ensuing months.

Third Month

Feels self conscious . . . people can read his thoughts . . . has strong feelings about some of the things we've been talking about . . . his relapse at his University was due in part to his not being ready to see Professor U (the colleague whom patient opposed prior to his breakdown) hears people talking about Felicia . . . it's very annoying . . . saying critical things that it is strange that a married woman comes to visit him . . . his parents wouldn't let him ride a bicycle until it was too late . . . he doesn't like to say critical things about his parents . . . it's very tiring to him but he knows it has to be done.

He says, "I feel ashamed I haven't realized how sick I've been. Finding that letter from Judith (in which she told him she would not marry him) was one of the grimmest moments in my life. I have a good deal of fear, and it has to do with women . . . This is very tiring for me to talk about." (He clearly is experiencing intense anxiety at this point.) He knows more, but is not ready yet to talk about it. He's had about all he can take for today. . . . We end the session at that point.

He says,"I am very much bothered by the talking I hear. Today I kept hearing people say that Felicia was here, but this seemed very unlikely to me". (Felicia was a friend who came to the hospital to visit Professor Marsh. She was the former wife of a colleague.) It is clear he felt intense guilt at seeing her, and that he projected his guilt onto other patients on his floor in the hospital. The projection of his guilt became an illusion to him, impairing his perception of reality and showing the tenuousness of his hold. And why did he feel so guilty?

The next day he says, "I feel much calmer. This is the result of our talk yesterday, about my feelings toward Felicia and my sense of guilt about this . . . about my mother . . . fear of hurting her feelings . . . I think I must live a gayer life . . . being alone too long has a lot to do with my illness. It was a mistake to have lived at my parents' home while I was at M.I.T. I didn't have enough sense to know this. I should have moved out. I was afraid doing so would have hurt their feelings."

The above suggests that Professor Marsh has urgent needs for maternal interaction. He still depends on his mother to meet these, but he now seeks interaction from other women. But to seek other women would hurt his mother's feelings and thus evoking guilt. It is noteworthy the guilt is for hurting his mother's feelings, not for engaging in incestuous sex, as might be expected according to conventional psychoanalytic theory.

Feels it's imperative he see his mother in the light of what we've been talking about . . . surprised to find how helpful it is to talk to me the way he does. . . . I say your mother is endearing and that evokes a desire to protect her. It would be difficult to get angry at her. He does not get angry with her, he replies.

Parents visit patient, first visit by his mother.

Following the first visit with his mother Professor Marsh did not comment to me about how the visit went, or how he appraised the accuracy of what we had been saying. However I saw her and asked her how he seemed to her. She said "He has a tan. I am glad of that because I heard he had been confined". I asked, "Did he seem himself?" "Yes," she said, "I saw no evidence of illness, except he said if we had no objection he would get a light for his cigarette."

Her comment, her first comment to me, that he had a " tan,"

seemed odd to me. It did show interest and concern for him, but seemed focused on superficial externals rather than sensitivity to his internal experience. This is borne out by her comment she sees no evidence of illness, (though he was psychotic at the time). I began to see why he could not talk to her. I found it difficult to talk to her myself. Her comment about his asking permission to light a cigarette does suggest awareness of autonomy in their interaction, but that his asking for permission was unusual for him. I guess asking for permission was part of his testing the accuracy of what we had been talking about concerning his mother.

Sense of aloneness . . . does most things alone . . . in Paris he would go see someone about every second or third day, rest of the time would be alone . . . very few people who mean much to him or with whom he feels comfortable. . . . He enjoys talking to me there's no question about that.

Feels more on his feet . . . perhaps because of the things we have been talking about . . . feels a number of things have become clear to him

Did he tell me the University has informed him of his increase of salary?

Feels strongly that Felicia is good for him

Fourth month

Thinks his standard defense against loneliness was engrossing his mind in physics . . . wants to keep his mind relaxed for several months. I say it will be six months before he is ready for strain.

He's surprised to realize the extent to which his relations with his mother have influenced his life . . . assumes influenced his relations with other women, also.

Hopes I had a good weekend. . . . Well, he had a very good weekend . . . actually did go to his University Sunday . . .

spent a few hours listening to music and sitting around. I ask, in Felicia's apartment? Yes, he says and then stopped in his apartment to pick up clothes.. Last time he was in his University he was still loused up . . . still trying to believe he was not mentally ill.

Still skating along . . . not much confidence . . . main difficulty he can't seem to get back to his work . . . and doesn't know how else to fill his time . . . does feel like seeing people and here doesn't have to force himself too much.

Hopes I had a good weekend. . . . Well, he had a very good weekend. Did both more and less than he expected. Professor U (the colleague he had opposed) was out of town so did not have to see him..

Has accepted the necessity for a gradual schedule of activities . . . hopes to move to the University next fall. . . .

Weekend went well. One day with his parents was enough . . . mother displayed affection to a degree he disliked, to the effect everyone she loved was under one roof. That's what she really liked . . . noticed a tendency of his parents to manage things to an extent he, himself, would find unacceptable.

"When my mother tells you to do something you end up doing it"

Further recognition of her power over him and his vulnerability to her power to control him. Here again was his conflict. He needed love but it took away his independence.

Sometime later he said, "I've concluded I'm a terrifically lonely person . . . find I can't seek out friends . . . tremendous relief when my parents phoned last night. Perhaps one of the big bases of my troubles is that I have remained too dependent on my parents."

And of course he is correct. He is too dependent on them.

They enrage him, they drive him crazy, yet he feels "tremendous relief' when they phone. Why? Because he needs to interact with someone, he can count on them. He does need to talk to someone. A person's sanity depends on social interaction. Without anyone to talk to he will go insane. So he exists in a double bind, he must interact with people yet interacting endangers his sanity.

"What is the purpose of women? How does one get strength from them?" This question, asked in the context of his undue dependence on his mother, suggests why he had not developed adequate relations with other women. He could not obtain "strength" from a woman because he behaved with them in the same way he did with his mother, by submitting to them, by foregoing his autonomy with them. By "strength" I believe he meant autonomy. He did not know how to relate to a woman autonomously, as a person with opinions and a will of his own. His experience led him to believe this was impossible.

Is so dependent on me. . . feels weak to be so dependent. . . . Seems to him he has to take hold of himself and get along in life. Is it all right to not be productive for a while? Yes, it is all right, I reply.

Fifth month

Says he sits on the floor for hours at a time waiting for something to happen . . . feels he could teach a course to under graduates the way he is right now.

He's decided he better be more frank with me . . . expects I'll think less of him. . . . He's slept with eight women in his life . . . all but one he feels all right about.

He was very poor at doing things as a boy . . . his father never played . . . worked all the time . . . never taught him to, did teach him multiplication tables.

Sitting playing bridge with three pretty nurses . . . feeling

desperate . . . losing his image as a professor . . . pleading for something to be done.

I have interview with Felicia . . . a pretty woman . . . dark eyes. red tender mouth, great figure, quiet, intense, asks why I don't give Professor Marsh electroshock . . . I ask, is she trying to convince me? Does she have confidence in me? She says that sounds like a threat. It is a threat, I reply, and if she continues to urge to him seek electroshock, I will try to persuade him to stop seeing her.

Says he needs some gaiety.

Seventh Month I was away on vacation.

Eighth month

"Feels he's lying down on the job . . . should go back to his University and succeed. Should be trying harder.

Starts to leave my office, turns around and shakes my hand.

He's becoming friendlier, he is less afraid I will control him.

"I was not allowed to ride a bicycle until I was a senior in high school. I was hopeless at sports, always slow running, couldn't catch a ball. Still can't catch a fly-ball. If I caught one it would be pure coincidence. I have no eye-hand coordination."

Professor Marsh lacked control of his own body, a form of autonomy deficiency which contributed to doubts about his ability to control other human functions. Forbidden to ride a bicycle, he was probably discouraged from doing many other boyhood things such as run, climb, jump, wrestle or throw a ball. This was verified subsequently. Both parents were sedentary people, unathletic, and apprehensive about physical activity. Professor Marsh's father was also unable to throw a ball and never played catch with his son.

Below is a drawing of a human figure done at my request at this time.

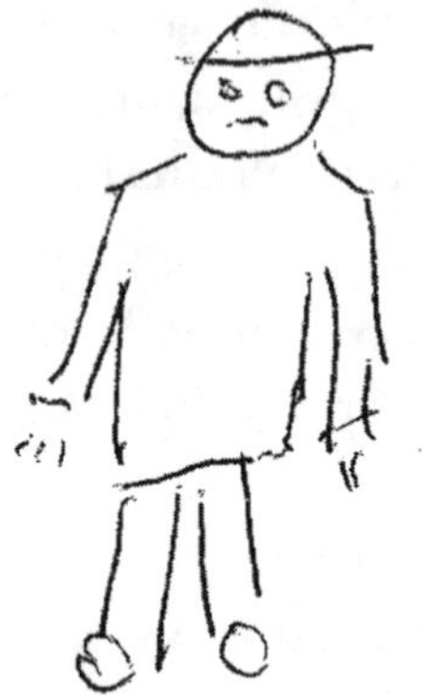

This drawing is weird in its sharply limited conceptualization of anatomy and feelings. It indicated a severely impaired ego structure and function. It made more understandable his uncertainty about himself and his inability to stand up to his mother, or people in general.

He says, "At times I was angry at my parents and I hid out in my room. I don't have many feelings. I mean, can a person be angry and not realize it? What kind of things would a person be angry at and not know it?"

Professor Marsh's unconscious anger was becoming conscious. Loss of one's autonomy to another person arouses the most intense anxiety and rage. Believing he could not survive a confrontation, Professor Marsh as a child found he could deal with his fury at his dominating mother by withdrawing to his room. Later he repressed his rage, did not "have many feelings." No doubt other feelings besides rage—incestuous or whatever—would have proved equally unpopular with his mother and should also be repressed.

At camp he couldn't hike as well as the other boys . . . at

first limped along behind . . . was very determined to catch up.

The way he leans on Felicia has changed . . . the thrill no longer is there.

He was resenting her control over him.

Last night he enjoyed himself at the dance,

but can enjoy himself with other women?

He doesn't know how to spend his time from hour to hour or even for months or years . . . he's all right when he's with someone, there he's all right.

Kissed a girl one time and she cried, said she had tried to be fond of him, but liked someone else.

This experience hardly increased confidence in his love making abilities.

Ninth month, November

Which is the cart and which the horse, getting stuck in physics or difficulty with people?

Felicia tells him he should be struggling more. I ask him what he thinks? He says he feels like struggling very little. I say, I advise him to struggle very little.

My focus is on what he thinks, rather than what Felicia or I think.

Cathy (the woman he had been close to for seven years) said he was so interested in physics there wasn't enough else for her to talk to him about.

A helpless lover.

Tenth month, December

He has great respect for people who are able to get along.This is a change in his thinking. He used to take that for granted. . . . Research in physics is achieved only by an agony of effort.

The only place he feels alive is with me. I ask why? He

replies with me he feels he can talk about what concerns him.

Because I reward his talking

He's puzzled about his relations with Felicia, she always seems to be pushing him to try harder. I say, I always tell him the opposite.

Felicia keeps trying to control him. I urge him to oppose her.

He does talk about personal things far more than he used to

Tried to do some physics yesterday for a couple of hours. I ask if he felt interested? Yes, he says, he awoke this morning working on some problems in physics.

There are few people he likes.

Eleventh month January.

Physics is a man's subject.

He thinks that the long struggle for independence with his parents was one reason he didn't tell them more, that to do so threatened his independence. Talking with me is different. I seem more impersonal.

By impersonal he means I consider his opinions objectively. I do not try to control what he thinks.

Second year. During the following months he repeated the following themes.

Still doesn't feel better.

"Is it all right if I just go back and lie down?" I reply, "It certainly is all right."

He doesn't see how he can gain strength, doesn't see how he can gain strength without doing something. I say he can gain strength from talking to me.

I reward his thinking rather than control it.

Patient's mother tells me she has a conviction her son's stay in the hospital is weakening him . . . that he is not trying hard enough. She favors moving him to a less comfortable part of

the hospital. There he won't like the hospital so much and will try harder to get out. She anticipates his visit home as her opportunity to make him try harder.

Both his mother and Felicia, the two women he depends on for love, keep trying to control his thinking, keep telling him his thinking is wrong.

Professor Marsh says his desire to live isn't very strong. "You survive because your parents expect you to."

No wonder he isn't eager to live. He doesn't live because he wants to.

I keep telling him to do what he wants.

Meaning he can control what he thinks and does.

September

He didn't want to go to M.I.T. because he didn't want to live in the same city as his parents. In another city he would feel his private life was more his own.

October

He says, "I used to fight with my father about some things."

He was confident enough of his opinions to argue with his father.

November

Had a pretty good time. Alicia cooked supper for him. The seminar went all right (He is now giving seminars on physics for graduate students and faculty at a nearby college [not his own University]).

Professor Marsh has struck up a friendship with a patient named Jane. He is feeling close to her because she seems to understand how he feels, much more than Felicia does. He says, "I'm not very close to my parents. I don't think my mother ever understood very much about anything I felt or

thought." He adds, "It's not her fault. I was a difficult boy for a person like her to bring up."

Again, Professor Marsh was showing steadily increasing insight into his dynamics. His relationship with Jane shows an increasing social competence. He may be able to find a replacement for Felicia and for his mother. Then he will be able to resolve his autonomy conflict—which I believe must happen for everybody in order to become an adult.

In another session, Professor March tells me, "Physicists are difficult to be married to. At parties they either talk physics, which women can't understand, or say nothing."

December

Early in his stay in the hospital his parents had moved from their home in Massachusetts and were living nearby. He tells me, "I wouldn't say my parents have been zero help. In certain ways its been nice to have them around." My mother amuses me some times. She looks as though she wants to do something to please me, but all she can think of is perhaps discussing what kind of pie I like, or folding my socks in a certain way". . . . His mother does not reveal her thoughts and feelings, does not show whether she really likes something.

Being "amused" by his mother's behavior indicated increasing objectivity and autonomy, a dramatic change from his earlier reactions of uncontrollable fear and rage at her misperceptions of him. He was no longer confused because he had come to understand that she was mistaken. So his identity was becoming more secure. He was growing up.

Again he talks about his lack of people he can feel close to, and how few people understand the world of physics. He feels lucky he met me, somebody he can talk to.

I believe that he will find there are many people out in the world who will "talk" with him as I do, not the way his mother does.

Professor Marsh's amazement stemmed from the newness of an interaction which strengthened him, and the realization of how much he needed social relationships. Never realizing that there was a remedy for his loneliness, he had always proceeded on the premise that he must get along alone.

"I guess I could go on quite a while the way things are, But they still aren't good." I ask, "What's missing?" He answers, "Being able to move around, and the thing I'm always talking about, someone to be close to. I don't have much confidence in ever finding one." He then returns to a familiar theme: The woman would have to be much more understanding than his mother, who hardly knows him at all.

Clearly, he still had a way to go to get well.

It's so unnatural for him to seek people out, so unlike his field of physics, he doesn't know how to solve such a problem.

Professor Marsh's parents are moving back to Massachusetts tomorrow. He says that in some ways having them here has been helpful, but adds that "their way of doing certain things gets to me a little." I suggest that it gets to him a lot. Professor Marsh smiles. "Well, yes. Such as making a big deal of things that don't matter. For example, they shop around for groceries to get items a few cents cheaper and then talk about it, implying that he should do likewise."

His parents' willingness to relocate to be near their son showed their devotion. It explained why he depended on them. But they were only near him geographically, not psychologically.

Says he glares at people, is hypervigilant.

They threatened his ego, his identity, and he had to be always watchful to defend it.

November

It was nice seeing his parents. His mother again expressed the opinion he should engage in positive thinking (patient gives a little smile as he says this). . . . She will tell him to put on his rubbers. Yesterday for instance she told him he should wear an overcoat. Well he didn't. He thinks these comments by his mother probably do not affect him now. Rather long ago things were said which affected him, but which he cannot remember now.

This was a definitive, measurable turning point in treatment He at last dared take the radical step: disobeying a direct command of his mother.

December

Almost two years in the hospital, much improved and commuting to his University to teach part time and to see Alicia. He says he doesn't know what he needs to get well. He says that "need" means what he needs from other people. The very idea is a new orientation. He thought he needed things from people in order to be happy, but not to keep functioning. He said he doesn't like the word "need." He always wanted to be independent. He was quite touchy on the subject with his parents for a number of years. He didn't like to tell his parents things. He would never tell them about Judith, for example. Why not, I ask? "The fear they would make up my mind," he replies.

This statement supports the idea that the danger from his parents is their threat to his autonomy because they will make up his mind for him. He wants to make up his own mind. But he is unable to oppose them.

Says he wouldn't have gone into physics if he hadn't gone in the army; in the army there wasn't much his parents could do to run his life.

When he's seeing me he doesn't feel he should be doing

something else.

Third Year

Professor Marsh returned to his University and began seeing me as an out-patient, three 50-minute sessions a week, a schedule which lasted for several years, and less frequently for several more years.

"My parents keep annoying me. They don't mean to." Yesterday they talked about a sermon they'd just heard in church, and said that he would have enjoyed it. He announces, "I can stick it out just so long and then I leave. And once I've decided, I don't fool around."

He loaned his car to Felicia the other day. I ask why? "I couldn't say no." he replied.

Discussing the security he feels within his profession, he tells me, "A problem in physics is always there. If you reach an impasse you can set it aside and return to it a year later. People aren't that way." His example was Margie, the woman he was engaged to years ago. Now, if he wanted to find her, he could not. But he can reach any physicist in the world in less than an hour. "I can count on physics and physicists," he says.

Professor Marsh tells me that Felicia's habitual lateness is increasingly annoying. Kept waiting endlessly, he is feeling "pushed around." He is "getting tired" of being so helpless and submissive. On Sunday she phoned at 4:00 to say she couldn't make it to supper. By that time he had turned down another invitation. But Professor Marsh is still fond of Felicia, though he says, "I'm pretty fed up with her. I'm not ready yet to junk the whole thing, but I've come pretty close."

So Professor Marsh continued to have a conflict between autonomy and "love."

I ask how dependent on her he is? Could he do his work

without her? He says, "It seems to me that's what I've been doing, getting along without her. Is it surprising that I'm upset?" I say that I'm not the least surprised. He would like to depend on Felicia, but she keeps making him doubt his attractiveness, doubt himself.

Enjoyed seeing his parents yesterday. Talked to them a fair amount, more than usual. You can discuss things with my father, but not with my mother. Well, for example she thinks a good deal of the world is hostile to the U.S. and we should get out of the U.N. Another example is that labor unions are bad and should be abolished.

We talk about his surprise that he has come to depend on interaction with me—whereas to me it is perfectly natural.

Working on physics with colleagues. (Shows me four pages of mathematical physics he's just written.) Says it was a relief to find he can still do some physics that X and Y—senior professors of physics at his University—can't do.

"I sort of look forward to that." To what?" I ask? "To a chance to talk." "To whom?" I ask. "To you," he replies. I say, "I thought that's what you meant. I do, too."

During extended treatment Professor Marsh learned how to please as well oppose people. Instead of an aloof glare, he appeared friendly. His clothes became brighter. He smiled more, became warmer. When leaving a session, he would say, "Bye-Bye. Take care." He never did marry. However, he developed a close relationship with one woman, and then, after a period, with another. He continued his work at the forefront of theoretical physics. For his 60th birthday his colleagues, many from all over the world, presented him with a volume of articles written in his honor. More than seventy colleagues attended the ceremony.

Chapter Five
Elinor, The Head Down Girl

In the fall of her sophomore year at college Elinor had phoned her parents saying she was very upset, and she threatened suicide. She was told to come home and was brought to me for treatment

Elinor sits facing me in my office, her head bowed. Her posture is frozen, her face expressionless, withdrawn. Except for fleeting glances, eye-contact is almost entirely absent. Her hair, cut below her shoulders, falls over her face, almost hiding it. She wears jeans and is clean and neat. She talks in a low voice, clearly and urgently. She has thick glasses, buck teeth and a shortened upper lip so that her mouth barely closes, resulting in a slight lisp. Her appearance is weird, repels interaction and suggests major psycho-pathology.

She tells me, "My main trouble is sexual arousal." She says that it started two years ago during her sophomore year at Princeton. It has gradually increased and now completely dominates her life. The story behind it: She was away at boarding school for five years and had no friends. The girls were into drugs. Her only friend was a male instructor. Her first contact with boys was in college at Princeton where the sexual arousal began. She was interested in her academic courses, but because of her sexual arousal she felt unable to continue classes and took a year off, living at home. She says, "I hid in my room"—

feeling like a prisoner of her sexual symptoms which are still present and have been confirmed by a gynecologist.

I noted that she cited an authority to validate her sexual arousal. Could she not depend on her own perceptions?

Elinor says that the physical arousal is not accompanied by sexual desires. I ask what she means by sexual arousal. She describes moistness in her vagina and erection of her nipples and says she relieves herself by masturbating.

Such arousal without accompanying sexual feelings was pathological; as was her frankness.

She continues, "I had a love affair from across the lecture room, mainly by eye-contact. I never talked to him. I felt a wall inside myself. I had another love affair, without touch. Then I had sexual intercourse two or three times as an experiment. But it was extremely unsatisfactory."

She claims that other people could detect her sexual arousal and were disturbed by it. I ask how they detected it. "I'm not sure," she replies. "Maybe by heat given off by my body." In college she isolated herself in classrooms and in lunchrooms. "I know men were aroused by me because they had erections," she says. "I saw them and it made me nervous which made others nervous."

I question her again about people detecting her arousal. She answers, "I probably read more significance into what I saw than was warranted."

So Elinor backed off from opposing me.

Two weeks before this first meeting, she had been evaluated twice by another psychiatrist and assigned to treatment once a week, but had only one session before coming home. She felt that talking about her difficulties only increased the symptoms. She now thinks she should withdraw from college and

engage in treatment, either living at home or in a hospital. But her grandmother, parents and sister live at home. "They don't believe I'm ill," she says, and adds somewhat bitterly, "I asked my parents for treatment a year and a half ago, but they refused.

Her complaint—physical arousal without sexual desire—was bizarre. Her belief that people detected her arousal was probably an illusion, projection of her own thoughts—so-called ideas of reference. Such abnormal cognition suggested psychotic impairment of ego function. Why did she emphasize her family's disbelief of her illness? I wondered if her symptoms were a means to oppose her parents' claim she was not ill. Seeking treatment on her own at college was an act of independence and defiance.

Elinor was unsure of her own thinking, she could not believe something unless her parents agreed. She feared they were right and that she was wrong. My patient Leslie had the same difficulty convincing her parents that she needed help. When Professor Marsh's mother visited him in the hospital, her primary reaction was, "He had a tan," in effect denying the reality of his mental illness. I did not oppose Elinor's version of events, thus aligning myself on her side against her parents.

At this time, because of constraints in my schedule, I could not have regular individual sessions with Elinor. Instead she was seen by a colleague, Doctor M., three times a week as an out-patient. The clinical sessions presented here are family therapy conducted by me. They were held weekly and extended over a year.

The story of her treatment will trace her steady improvement as she gains confidence in her own thinking and increasingly opposes each family member.

In our initial family session Elinor's mother, a very neatly

dressed woman of faded prettiness, sat off to one side. Elinor's father, a small, tight-faced, articulate man, sat in the principle chair, facing me. When I told them what their daughter had said, the mother interjected, "Elinor really did have friends."

I noted she contradicted the patient. This was an autonomy conflict because the issue was who was right. Her mother clearly believed Elinor was wrong. Could Elinor believe she, herself, was right unless her mother agreed with her?

Elinor's mother continues, "We now believe she is ill and needs treatment."

Well, Elinor had won this one.

Later in the session, her father mentions her "disastrous" year at Princeton. He referred to her poor academic marks at college. Elinor's mother protested, "She got C's and B's." Her father responded: "I am a Princeton man!"

So C's and B's did not meet his standards. He sounded pompous.

In the next session with the parents, the mother tells me that she, herself, was an only child. Moreover, Elinor's grandmother, who is living at their home, is an only child and an early orphan. Elinor's father explains that he was distant with his mother and brother. Now he has few friends, and they rarely have guests in the house. "Our life is devoted to Elinor and her sister Beth," he says. "Perhaps we have been too possessive".

Both parents were neglected in *their* childhoods and had limited capacity to gain attention and affection from their peers. This impelled them to rely primarily on their children to fulfill their needs, a reversal of roles.

Later in the session the father remembers, "When Elinor first told us of the smell from her sexual arousal, I said "ridiculous."

The father's reaction to Elinor's symptoms was highly

relevant. At first glance her statement did seem ridiculous. But he was denigrating her thinking process.

He continues, "It would be very difficult to convince me that she should be put in a hospital, that she is that sick and it is my fault, and most difficult to convince me that she should be taken away from us."

This statement seemed to confirm that the father needed his daughter, and that he tended to place his needs before hers, ignoring her autonomy. He said "put" her in a hospital, which ignored her own opinion and implied that he would make the decision. Also, her father, although now acknowledging that Elinor was ill, denied any responsibility for causing her condition.

During a session alone with Elinor's mother, she says, "I haven't been able to see any family tensions which could have caused a nervous breakdown in one of our children."

She was very frightened that there might be truth in Elinor's accusations that they, as parents, had caused her breakdown.

She went on to say, "I saw a personality change in Elinor at age 14 following defeat in competition at school for editorship of the school paper, and for hockey captain. After that she was much more shy and self conscious. Elinor always had a very private life, but we never saw this as evidence of psychological difficulty."

Her defensiveness seemed to have blinded her to Elinor's inner turmoil through a lifetime.

An early December meeting with both parents: Her father begins by saying in a challenging voice, "We want to know the purpose of this meeting. The main thing we are feeling is frustration. We can't find a cause of the illness in our family, don't understand the treatment, don't understand what we can do to help."

Angrily opposing me, he is frightened that he might be wrong.

I reply that the purpose of the meeting is for me to attempt to answer all their questions—and I give them a copy of Theodore Lidz's little book, *The Origins and Treatment of Schizophrenia*.[43] I opposed Elinor's father, invoking other authority to support my opinion.

Later in the session Elinor's mother says, "Elinor and I were arguing about clothes, and afterwards Elinor apologized and said I had been right. The arguing isn't new, but the apology is." Her father comments that she and Elinor are black and white people. He is gray.

The implication by her mother was that Elinor should have apologized. But I wondered if she, the mother, might appropriately have also have apologized. Apparently the father thought so, too, though he quickly exonerated himself.

Dependent, authoritarian people—like Elinor's father—are often raised in families where discussion is unknown. They are incapable of compromise. As children, to preserve their sanity they have to find some way to oppose their parents. They do this by finding issues which represent their identity. For these they would do or die, i.e., risk loss of love and support. Giving in on symbolic issues means giving up autonomy and thus sanity. When such issues are involved, since they cannot give in to their parents, they cannot give in to anybody.

A meeting with Elinor's parents: He begins by saying that the Lidz's book on schizophrenia is very painful. He is now convinced that Elinor has schizophrenia. She has the symptoms the book described. He is convinced, too, that schizophrenia derives from family troubles caused by the fact that Elinor essentially had two mothers. He and his wife had been

married just one year and their older daughter Beth was two months when the grandmother moved into the house. She seemed unable to live alone and too shy to make friends.

He tells me Elinor's mother had serious fatigue when their first daughter, Beth, was born. The baby cried every two hours and had to be fed one ounce of milk. When Elinor was born, mother and grandmother decided to share her care, one week on, one week off. So she had two mothers. Beth, the older sister, reacted by being very shy, not wanting to grow up, not wanting to copy her own mother in such skills as cooking or knitting. The grandmother lived vicariously through the girls.

I say that his theory makes good sense to me. Two mothers would cause confusion in the choice of which model to follow. I ask Elinor's mother what she thinks about this theory. It makes sense to her, she replies.

It did make sense. It also exonerated her father from blame and distributed the responsibility between mother and grandmother. I was eager to agree to the theory in order to reward the father's highly intelligent and useful theorizing and his acceptance of parental etiological involvement, even if he did have to leave himself out of it.

We consider why Elinor does not talk to her parents. Her father says, "I think it's a fear of hurting our feelings by blaming us." I answer, "Perhaps," and say that Doctor M. suggests another reason: danger of losing her identity because her father does not believe her.

Dr. M. agreed with me that control of a child by parents may cause loss of identity.

A meeting in late December with Elinor's father and mother and including for the first time her grandmother. The grandmother says, "I think it would be a good idea to meet

with the whole family and bring things out in the open. Elinor is feeling sorry for herself. She takes a superior position intellectually toward the whole family, and toward everybody. She is very shy and thinks people will laugh at her." The grandmother adds, "Elinor always is for the underprivileged. I think Doctor M. should get Elinor to think "positively."

In the grandmother's view, bringing things out in the open at a family meeting would reveal the wrongness of Elinor's thinking and force her to think more "positively." The grandmother thought she knew better than Elinor or Doctor M. what was right and what was wrong, and would not hesitate to say so. Of course, telling Elinor her thinking was wrong would invalidate her thinking, particularly if that had been the pattern throughout her childhood. Certainly, Elinor would not be encouraged to reveal her thoughts to her grandmother or to anyone else. And yet, the grandmother seemed fond of her and concerned.

I then oppose the grandmother. I ask her "Are you shy?" She says that, yes, she is. I ask what made her shy. She answers, "Well, I was left an orphan at age two and until age five lived with seven different families. Then I stayed with one family."

She continues, "I think Elinor is reluctant to tell the family her troubles because she's ashamed of having fallen behind in her studies." She adds, "I think Elinor reads too much; it takes her away from people."

In mid-January the first full family meeting: present are Elinor, her mother and father, Beth, and her grandmother. The father says, "I dislike contention."

Elinor says angrily, "I think the family does suppress thoughts that are unpleasant." Her grandmother says, "Who put that thought in your head?" Elinor sarcastically mimics her:

"Who put that thought in your head?" Then she points at her grandmother and says accusingly, "You do that all the time!"

Elinor's ability to oppose her grandmother, to express resentment toward her in the presence of her family was new and a result of treatment.

She says, "I feel a pressure, mostly from my father, and it is killing me. His mere physical presence . . . and it's increasing.

What did she mean? Killing her ego? Her identity?

In late January, a meeting with mother and daughter. Elinor says, "My father has made me feel that most everything I have to say is ridiculous. When I try to write, I find I cannot. I've realized that the reason is I see my father standing looking over my shoulder, telling me that what I intend to write is ridiculous."

I believed that Elinor was correct, that she had internalized his constant put-downs and saw them as authoritative. Her father is telling her, not only that she cannot write, but also that she has a mind that produces ridiculous thoughts.

But her words were even more revealing about him than about herself. He, too, had deep doubts about his judgment, so that, like his daughter, being right was a measure of sanity. He had his own syndrome of control or be controlled, his own misgivings that Elinor might overwhelm him.

During this session, Elinor describes her father's "pronouncements" and calls them "authoritarianism."

She was becoming able to judge her father's opinion and to question its validity. I supported her.

I commented that he sounded authoritative to me also, and that he seemed completely unaware of it.

I ask Elinor, "What effect did your father's authoritativeness have on Beth?" She replies, "Beth has never had an opinion

different from her father's." I ask what effect that had on her mother. Elinor answers, "She couldn't see it. It's impossible for my mother to see any fault in my father."

She was gaining enough detachment to appraise the family dynamics in regard to autonomy.

In a family meeting in early February we take up the issue of the father's authoritativeness. He says, "I don't think I am authoritarian, but I can see how Elinor might have thought so." He says that his wife and mother-in-law believed that their role as women requires them to defer to him as the decision-maker. Elinor smiles. I ask her why. She answers: "Because he's off the point."

Here Elinor openly challenged her father. I noted his defensiveness, attributing any belief he was authoritarian to misperception by others.

A little later Elinor's father says, "I disapprove of premarital and extra-marital sex." I challenge him: "Do you see yourself as authoritarian on this issue?" Her father: "Well I guess I'm one of the few people left who see it that way. I do think the world would be much better off if more people agreed with me."

So sex raised its ugly head, another key issue on which Elinor and her family disagree. I noted that when considering whether he was authoritarian, her father chose sex to acknowledge that possibility. Almost certainly Elinor's sexual arousal was a reaction to her father's condemnation of sexuality. And why was he so emphatic on the subject? Did he protest too much? Was he disturbed by guilt over his own sexuality?

Unconscious dynamics were breaking out into the open. It did seem highly therapeutic for Elinor. The pressure from her family's constant disagreement with her opinions endangered her ego function. But her growing capacity to see that her family's thinking might be wrong could enable her to survive in that environment.

Elinor continues: "In the presence of my father I feel crushed." She goes on to say that most of the pressure comes from her father's perfectionism, and explains that "I'm a poor musician, but I love to play the piano. The other day I was playing away. Father came home. He began whistling the tune, but in the correct time." He interrupts: "I was teasing." She answers, "I wasn't even trying to play in correct time." He answers, "I'm such a terrible perfectionist. I even had a terrible time raking leaves as a boy."

I ask Elinor, "Do you feel like screaming right now?" "Yes," she says. "Every time during the session when I smile, I feel like screaming."

She saw the disastrous results of her father's perfectionism imposed on her mind through her lifetime. I noted that she said "crushed" by her father immediately after he acknowledged being authoritative about sex. What was the connection between being "crushed" and sex?

Elinor's father: "On Thursdays, Elinor has both a session with Doctor M. and this family session. Isn't it perhaps too much for her?" Elinor stands up and looks directly at him. Her voice full of anger, she says, "Can't you let me decide that for myself? I'm certainly able to decide whether it's too tiring and saying so!"

She rightly felt insulted that her father considered her so helpless, so weak, that she could not make that decision for herself. Her anger showed that she still could not discount his opinion. Moreover, she was increasingly aware of the harm caused by his pattern of depreciating her cognition.

After the session, I learned from him that two meetings in a day caused him considerable transportation problems.

So she also had sensed hypocrisy on his part, pretending his concern was for her.

When parents make decisions for children, they often do not see that they are damaging the children's judgment. They believe they are merely showing love, and see the resulting resentment as ingratitude.

Session in mid-February with Elinor and her parents: She recounted an episode when she and her friends were jumping on her bed. She remembers, "My father came in and yelled at me to stop that! Well that made me feel I wasn't allowed to have any friends." Her father replies, "I don't think children should jump on beds."

Many parents would permit bed-jumping, if not overdone. His prohibition against bed jumping was law in her father's mind, and dictums had to be enforced no matter what the consequences.

Elinor goes on to say, "I never had an allowance. I don't have a cent of my own right now. I'm told if I want money I just have to ask for it."

To have no money of her own, and be forced to ask for it, induced a sense of helplessness and dependence.

Later in the session her father says, "I hate pierced ears". Elinor asks, "Are you afraid of my ideas because they're so different?"

The issue had relatively little to do with ears and a lot to do with such questions as whose ears are they? Who had the right to decide about their piercing? Who was going to give in? Elinor extended the issue by proposing that any independent thinking would frighten and anger him.

At this point her mother intervenes, saying, "I think my husband is being unfairly accused." He says, "I agree. Yet there's no doubt that's the way I came across to Elinor."

Well, was he being unfairly accused? He sounded pretty authoritarian—and threatened by his daughter. Perhaps admitting he was wrong would mean to him his own brain was defective. His sanity was in as much danger as Elinor's. She was "crushing" him.

Why did her mother come to his rescue? Elinor had said her mother could not admit to any fault in him. This suggested a lack of autonomy on her mother's part, at least *vis-a-vis* her husband. Siding with him against Elinor further undermined her daughter's confidence.

Her father's comment that he might come across authoritarian lent therapeutic hope. But he exonerated himself from any responsibility by blaming Elinor. He claimed she just took what he said the wrong way.

Elinor says, "I feel crushed in my father's presence. He'd better stay away from me."

Not only was Elinor now raising her head, she was becoming belligerent and confrontational. Was she threatening her father? Again she used the word "crushed." This was a powerful word, meaning destroyed, annihilated. And what was being "crushed"? Her identity. Her autonomy. Her "self," even her sanity, her ability to think, to make decisions, to conduct her life, to take care of herself, to become an adult.

Her principle pathology was contained in her use of that word. It also suggested the effective focus of treatment, namely to protect and foster her ego.

Although Elinor was psychotic, her pathology occurs in most categories of mental disorder. Moreover, conflicts involving autonomy occur constantly between normal parents and children. Poor parents. We poor, well-meaning, loving parents, doing our best!"

A full family Meeting in early March: I say, "No one seems to be talking today." Elinor explains that she fears hurting members of her family by being critical or expressing anger. A little later I ask Elinor why she lowers her eyes. "To protect myself", she says. "If I look at them, I can't think. I get so self conscious."

Her thoughts were stalled by the danger of alienating her family, the danger of being disbelieved, of being considered silly. When I first saw Elinor, sitting with her head down, I thought the measure of her recovery would be the degree she raised her head as she talked to me, even though it must mean risking the loss of her wits.

Elinor later says, "When my grandmother told me to "snap out of it," I got angry and yelled at her. Elinor's parents agree that she is expressing her anger more. She continues, "My mother resents it when I tell her I know more about something than she does. And vice versa." Her mother identifies with this, saying "I have been fighting with my mother all my life." Her father interjects, "And they both think they're right!" Her mother says," After one fight with my mother I hid a small frying pan she liked to use." At the end of the session Elinor's father says, "Did you I notice I got off easy tonight?"

The family's ability to talk more freely and objectively—and less defensively—had increased astonishingly. This change, I believed, indicated major therapeutic improvement. Elinor's pathology was merely a part of the pathology of the entire family. Their increased ability to talk to each other provided all members with more support for the validity of their thoughts.

In a family meeting Elinor talks about the allowance she now receives. "I feel it would be despicable of me if I saved it," she says, "because that would be seeking independence."

This meant that seeking independence was despicable. So Elinor's struggle for autonomy—for survival—was condemned.

The answer from Elinor's father was not recorded.

Elinor reacts violently, shouting, "You're so self-righteous. I hate you! There, I've said it." She sobs quietly, then reaches for her mother's hand and lays her head on her mother's lap, keeping it there for several moments.

This was a turning point in treatment. Elinor changed from blaming herself to blaming her father for her insanity. Clearly, she still had a long way to go, but now she could understand that he was wrong to dismiss her thoughts as ridiculous. She was breaking free from his "crushing" domination. And it is noteworthy that she turned to her mother in an endearing way, hoping for reassurance at this point, and her mother did comfort her.

Again, her father's reaction was not recorded, but it must have been non-threatening to Elinor because shortly thereafter she continued her attack.

She angrily says, "Father wields the whip hand. He thinks he owns me. He's extremely possessive." She went on to describe herself sitting next to a boyfriend on the sofa. Her father came over and knelt against her leg. Her parents' reaction to what she had just said makes her answer, "You sound like broken records. It makes me feel you haven't heard what I've been saying."

Not hearing, not understanding, sent Elinor the message that she was crazy. Her father's act of kneeling against her leg seemed very intrusive and threatening to Elinor's identity. Also it was erotic. Sexually seductive behavior by her father must have been a cause of Elinor's symptom of sexual arousal.

After the session, when her father and I are alone, he asks me, "What does self-righteous mean?"

This question was almost unbelievably naive; he appeared sincere. He seemed unaware of the intrusiveness of his behavior. Because his own ego boundaries were unclear, he was confusing Elinor about her boundaries.

In mid-March during a session with mother and daughter, Elinor says that when she first received an allowance from her father, she immediately bought a pictorial history of the Civil War. But because neither of her parents seemed to understand why she wanted an allowance, she felt felt ungrateful and selfish.

Later in the session Elinor says, "I hate my father. I've lost all the respect I had for him, at least in his relationship with me. I don't love him now. I feel sorry for him. I think he's a nice man; it's just that with me . . . I was very angry at my mother, but am not now."

Elinor thinks she provoked her father in the last session, getting him to say things that would make her lose her temper and have the courage to tell him he was self-righteous and that she hated him. She continues, "What he was saying reminded me of what he said two years ago when I told him I was ill and asked for help and he ignored me. That's when I discovered that he could be wrong."

So she was gaining confidence in her cognition. She was beginning to understand that she could be right, even if her father disagreed with her. Therefore she realized her mind did not always produce silly thoughts. She had known she was ill and the chief evidence was the existence of sexual feelings—sensations she experienced whether her father believed her or not.

This may be a reason she had these symptoms, to establish her autonomy.

In a late March meeting with the full family, Elinor says, "I was not shocked at telling my father he was self-righteous and that I hated him. I'd known it for some time—and knew I would have to say it to his face to get well."

I believed she was correct. To establish her autonomy, she had to say these things out loud and prove to herself that she had a mind of her own.

She goes on to say, "Today I want to get into another area—my feelings about my sister. My parents may think this is a terrible thing to say, but I've come to realize I dislike Beth as a person. I think she dislikes me, even hates and loathes me." Elinor went on to describe a life-long rivalry for her father's approval.

Her mother says, "My husband and I do not think these thoughts are terrible."

So Elinor discovers that her parents did not always think she was wrong.

Elinor then says that she feels very strong pressure from her sister because of Beth's hostile attitude. I comment, "It appears your sister's attitude is impeding your recovery."

Beginning the next family session on the first of April, Elinor says, "I'll preface my statements by saying I'm quite upset tonight. We planned to have a family session at home and talk about the relationship between Beth and me. I was quite enthusiastic about that, but then on Saturday my mother asked, do I still want to—which put the whole responsibility on me. Then my mother said "Don't be too hard on Beth." Well, there you are, compounding my guilt. We finally went ahead last night for two hours, but I had to do it all myself, my parents just sat there.

Her father says angrily, "I think Elinor is being very unfair to us. I was eager to proceed with the conference, but then Elinor said she didn't want to. Later she said she did, as an emergency."

Elinor cries out, "I want my father to admit guilt!"

Very angrily, he shouts, "Well I don't feel guilt. I made a terrible mistake!" (Probably referring to his refusal to provide Elinor with treatment when she asked him for it two years ago.) He continues, "But it was the best decision I could make at the time. So how can I feel ignorant?" (Probably meaning guilty.)

I ask Elinor,"Why do you want him to admit guilt?" She answers that his failure to do so is preventing her from getting well.

She cannot believe she is right unless her father admits he is wrong—and feels guilty about it.

By assigning him power to judge her sanity, she has placed herself in a helpless position. Recovery will depend upon her gaining the ability to believe she is right when he believes she is wrong

Elinor was still a long way from being able to do this. And why did her father become so angry? Some people find it very difficult to admit error to themselves—and even more difficult to admit it to somebody else. For such people, being wrong means being defective or "ignorant," as Elinor's father put it.

At the end of this session Elinor's father tells me, "I don't see any progress and feel great frustration."

We were at a treatment impasse.

Elinor begins an early April family session by saying, "My father doesn't think in terms of difference." She describes a period of her life when she and her mother differed constantly. I point out that Elinor was developing autonomy by differing with her mother, a normal process in adolescent development.

Her father says that he himself never had such an experience. His grandfather died when his father was seventeen. His father then took on the role of supporting the family until the older siblings grew up, and did not marry until age thirty-seven. He was a silent man who rarely expressed his feelings, and uttered few opinions. Recently, he became disabled by a stroke, and Elinor's father visits him two or three times a week. They have become much closer and Elinor's father regrets their past remoteness.

By turning here to his own experience, he seemed to acknowledge the validity of his daughter's opposition. The fact that he had not experienced conflict with his father explained his difficulty in accepting the conflict between himself and Elinor.

Elinor asks him to tell about his mother. He says, "My mother was very talkative." He describes his father and brother and himself sitting silent at the dinner table while she talked and talked. She was adamantly against his marriage and, in fact, would have preferred him not to marry at all. She refused to visit him and Elinor's mother. "This hurt me a good deal," he remarks.

Elinor's mother says she considered her mother-in-law very selfish, so she supported her husband in his hurt. I comment that he must have felt very mixed up at this time. He answers, "Yes, quite." He thought that his wife was wrong about his mother—but now sees she was correct

I say I am struck by the similarities: Elinor's father was prevented from having autonomy—a life of his own—by his father's early death and the family's needs. His mother was possessive and hindered the development of his autonomy. Now Elinor is feeling that he is hindering her autonomy. I continue, "It seems possible that Elinor's father has not yet fully

developed his own autonomy, and that's why he is hindering it in Elinor."

Then I wonder aloud whether he can or should change so Elinor can get well. Can she recover in these surroundings? Since interacting with family has made the patient ill, home is frequently the most difficult place to get well. However, it may be the best place, if she can do it, since sooner or later she may want to function normally with her family. I say, "These are higher stakes." Her father says, "We all want her to shoot for the higher stakes." Elinor says, "I love my family and want to have them for a family." I say, "You all are making excellent progress, so we'll continue this way."

Later in the day Elinor's father phones and says that on the way home she announced that she needed to go to the hospital to get well. She also said that her mother hated her, which, of course, upset her mother. Then two nights later she more or less demanded that they send her to the hospital, telling her father that he owed it to her. I tell him that he should present the hospital as one alternative. She may be testing him. Whatever her decision, it should be respected. Her father asks how much the hospital will cost? I say $12,000 per month. He agrees to send her, if she insists.

I consulted with Doctor M. who has been seeing Elinor individually. She—Doctor M. was female—confirmed that Elinor strongly desired to enter the hospital, and she had been thinking independently that Elinor needed hospital care.

One reason was that Elinor's comments to her parents were causing tension between them which she could not stand. In particular, she was outraged at her mother's concern for the cost of treatment. Hospitalization was arranged for the following week.

Doctor M. phoned to say Elinor had changed her mind about going to the hospital now. Her reasons seemed OK. Her father phoned to cancel the session for tonight because of his wife's illness, and Elinor was apprehensive about driving alone with him.

I suggest a phone conference with him. He tells me that Elinor and her mother got into a "terrible exchange" about whether to tell friends and acquaintances she was in a mental hospital. I ask about the fight. One-sided, says her father, Elinor angry, her mother defending calmly. However, her mother was so exhausted by it, she lay down afterward. Then she contracted the flu. Also, she has been going through menopause and has been bleeding the last few weeks.

A pretty heavy implied responsibility for Elinor. It appeared, I feared, that current interactions between Elinor and her family, and between me and her family, had aroused anxieties which were beyond the family's capacity to handle.

In the next session Elinor says that an important reason she decided to stay home was the fact that in the hospital she would only see her parents once a week. Therefore, she would not have as much opportunity to express her anger at them. She knew this was hard on her mother, but it helped her.

Elinor thinks she's getting better, and her father agrees. They had celebrated Elinor's birthday and it was an enjoyable affair: cocktails, champagne, presents. Elinor was apparently relaxed and enjoying herself and more open with him than at any time heretofore. At the party she kept her head raised most of the time, and even engaged in occasional eye-contact.

This, indeed sounded like improvement. It confirmed that hiding her anger was one reason Elinor had kept her head down.

Late April family meeting: Since sex is an area where her

father acknowledged being authoritarian, I decide to bring it up at this point. I give my hypothesis that when Elinor feels that other people feel loathing for her sexual arousal, she is projecting her own loathing for her sexual desires. Elinor rejects this suggestion. I then ask Elinor's mother about her own attitude toward sex. She says that outside marriage, sex is unwise, wrong for her, but standards are personal. However, a promiscuous woman is worse than a woman who murders in passion. But she would accept Elinor living with a man, though she would try to talk her out of it. Elinor says she is surprised at the liberalness of her mother's view, though she doesn't believe it.

Wow! Elinor's mother said sexual promiscuity is worse than murder, at least passionate murder. So sex must be pretty bad in her eyes. "Loathsome?" In the face of such views, how could Elinor as a child believe her own emerging sexual urges were normal!

In childhood, a mother's response can be more important and have greater effect than all other consequences. "Don't run! You'll fall down!" Such frightened, angry cries from a mother, repeated often enough, may teach her child that the chief danger of falling down is not a bruised knee but to be shouted at by its mother. So the physical consequences of falling down may seem hardly relevant. The child may have never fallen down, never experienced that outcome. Though the consequences implied by the mother's shout may not be specific, the principle message is that the injury will be horrendous. It is to be avoided at all costs.

The resulting memories permanently influence the child's decisions, instilling confidence or lack of confidence. If the mother is not overly frightened by running and even pleased, the memory of running and falling and bruising a knee can enter the child's calculations. But if the primary memory is of the mother screaming, the child may never run, or run cautiously and therefore awkwardly.

Being shouted at can stun children, can frighten them out of their wits. They may literally lose their ability to think, at least temporarily. So the danger of falling down is extrapolated to losing their wits. In the extreme, the lesson may be to do nothing at all, except what has been approved in advance by their mother.

Elinor says that both parents think sex is loathsome. She believes that her sister, influenced by their parents, feels the same way.

Loathing must have been connected with Elinor's symptom of sexual arousal. Moreover, sex represented opposition to her parents. But, my goodness, the family had certainly arrived at a new level of discourse. Her father was able to think about family behavior which could have influenced Elinor's feelings about sex. And the level of anxiety in the family was not as intense as a few days ago.

In a session early in May, Elinor's father says that he was the primary person who changed Beth's diapers. Elinor's mother was an only child and had had no contact with children. When an infant of her own needed a diaper change, that was too much for her. She didn't know what to do.

Elinor remembers a time at the shore when her grandmother was taking a shower. Elinor approached the shower, not realizing she was in it. Both her grandmother and her mother cried out in alarm warning her to keep away. I say that this sounds like a good example of the way a child is taught an opinion about the non-acceptability of sex.

Elinor's father says, "I would find it difficult to continue a

relationship with a daughter if she became sexually promiscuous." He then seemed to contradict himself. He says, "I think we haven't found any incident that explains Elinor's symptom of sexual arousal, or feelings that sex is loathsome, or that the rest of us are repelled by sex.

Again, wow! Elinor's father said that promiscuous sex is so bad he would cut off relations with her. He was even more extreme than Elinor's mother. I, myself, was not strongly in favor of promiscuous sex, but these views did seem extreme. They explained Elinor's difficulty opposing her parents about the goodness or badness of sex. What a conflict for a daughter! Agree that sex is bad or be kicked out of the family.

But her father flatly rejected any possibility that he was a cause for his daughter's mental disorder and rejected Elinor's and my convictions. He thinks we are both silly. I wondered, "Is my hypothesis wrong?"

During a mid-May full family meeting, Elinor says she thinks she is going mad—and feels like screaming—when just sitting. The moment she talks, that feeling—perhaps rage—decreases. She now senses less pressure from her father, though it is still considerable and comes from men in general. The improvement is due to talking to her father. She now is able to converse with him—about Jimmy Carter, the Civil War. She initiates the conversations, asks him questions, because she really wants to know. I ask why she can't talk to men. Their prestige, she says, and the sex of men.

Elinor says that now when she drives, she no longer has the sensation of cars converging on her, which she did prior to taking stelazine (her medication).

So the drug does seems to be having a therapeutic effect.

Family meeting in early June, following the parents' return

from a trip to Europe: Her father says again, "I see effects, but no causes of Elinor's illness in the family." Elinor says, "I don't feel I am loathsome in any place except home. My mother thinks I'm loathsome because of my symptoms. The main person who thinks I'm loathsome is my sister. She thinks sex is disgusting, flirting is disgusting, and a woman chasing a man is disgusting. She will be at a dance and a man will approach her whom she very much wants to dance with, and she puts an expression on her face which says go away. My sister has done very little dating."

We learn that the onset of Elinor's symptoms came when she was strongly attracted to a very sexually attractive man—handsome, heavily muscled. Did she, like her sister, send out positive and also negative signals that said, "Don't touch me. If you touch me, you will hurt me."

Elinor's father says, "I'm a great flirter, I wink a lot." He then says, "Maybe I'm a little old fashioned about sex, but not enough to cause an illness. Have you given more thought to a physical exam?"

Elinor says she dreads a physical exam, hates being touched, hates doctors, hates her body being looked at. Being touched will hurt her. She cannot say why or in what way. I ask, "Is sex involved in touching?" She replies that dancing includes sex feelings, but she thinks that her sister Beth excludes them.

Elinor explains that she doesn't raise her eyes because looking at female breasts and male genitals causes intense embarrassment. It is not fear of eye-contact. She tells us that Doctor M. says her preoccupation with sex organs is because of a desire to be held. That makes good sense to her.

I'm not sure it makes good sense to me.

Elinor says that with her mother she senses a mutual put-down. She realizes that this may be projection, attributing to her mother the attitude in her own head. A kind of rivalry. She will not accord to her mother the same attention she will her father. She has the sense that her mother withdraws attention and gives perfunctory answers while reading a magazine.

Her mother answers that she is unaware of this and is shocked that Elinor feels it. Elinor replies that she is certain that keeping her eyelids down is related to something fundamental in their relationship. She feels her mother hates her because she is a rival for her father's affection. I ask if she sees anything sexual in this. She says no. I ask, "When did this rivalry start?" She answers that it started when she began having her sexual symptoms.

This was very different from autonomy conflict. It was the first appearance of statements or behavior which related directly to Oedipal conflict. That this appears now requires a reappraisal of her psychodynamic pathology. Psychoanalytic concepts of psychosexual development of the child focus on infantile sexuality, in which the daughter, for example, competes with the mother for sexual union with the father. That such rivalry was central in the development of Elinor's autonomy seemed unlikely, yet the role of sexuality in her development remained unexplained.

In late June Doctor M. phones and says she recommends hospitalization. Elinor is now ready to do it for her own benefit. I phone her father who says, "We've gotten nowhere this way, so let's go ahead with hospitalization." He sees no improvement and no causes in family influence.

Were Elinor's father and mother blinded by the danger to their self-images?

Three days later Elinor was admitted to the hospital.

She and her parents visited me in my office. Elinor is trembling. She says she is petrified. I ask what made her decide to come in to the hospital. She says there was a conflict with her grandmother the other day in a store. They both behaved badly. Her grandmother insisted on buying material to make Elinor two dresses. Elinor did not want two. It was a battle of wills.

Again, autonomy conflict thrusts itself into the scene. But Elinor now seems able to engage in such battles with her grandmother, opposing her rather than submitting.

Significantly, this autonomy conflict with her grandmother led to Elinor's arrival in the hospital. This implied that she still felt *unable* to resolve such conflicts at home, and so must escape into the hospital.

I ask about the battle of wills. Elinor says her grandmother accused her of being selfish and of thinking of nobody but herself. When Elinor says "behaved badly," she means selfishly in not complying with her grandmother's wishes.

It was increasingly clear that living at home kept Elinor under pressure from frequent assaults on her ego. If she could have said no to her grandmother, and at the same time kept her self-esteem, she could have withstood her grandmother's wrath. But to accomplish this while living at home would be difficult.

At the end of June, after seven days, Elinor signed out of the hospital "against advice." The hospital record showed that Doctor B., the admitting physician, reported Elinor's attitude and behavior markedly changed. She was vigorous, open, with direct eye-contact. The nurses reported that Elinor principally secluded herself. She was pleasant to them when approached, but very superficial. The nurses report Elinor had appeared to receive messages over the T.V., though she denied having hallucinations.

The internist who examined Elinor reported there were no abnormal findings, except maldistribution of pubic hair. He recommended a gynecological consultation but he did not think endocrine levels would be abnormal.

I now wonder whether Elinor's testosterone blood level was elevated.

The only other abnormal finding was a tremor, which the internist attributed to anxiety. She told Dr. B. that she was leaving the hospital because she couldn't stand the other patients.

But in Doctor B.'s opinion, Elinor thought she wasn't crazy and didn't belong in a crazy hospital. My thought was that whatever the reasons for leaving the hospital, Elinor was doing what she wanted to do, even to the extent of opposing the hospital authority. This is why, I believe, she was "vigorous, and maintained direct eye-contact"

Family session the day after Elinor's departure from the hospital: She now plans to attend typing and shorthand school, and feels up to night courses at college. She felt immense obstacles to getting well in the hospital. All the patients were so depressed. She preferred facing her difficulties at home where she can master them.

Three weeks later, meeting alone, Elinor tells me that she can now easily discredit her grandmother's opinion—for example a disagreement over whether to close a window to protect her house plants. At first she had hoped her parents would recognize their authoritarianism and confirm it, validating her thinking. Now she realizes that this will never happen. She will have to trust her own judgment.

This shift away from validation by others was a key step toward recovery.

Her parents' view of people, Elinor says, is profoundly

different from hers. They blame their own behavior on others. She sees the real causes of their behavior. Moreover, she is for the underdog. They are for the overdog. Equating recovery with confidence in her own thinking, she sees that her best chance is to leave her family and live among people whose values are more like her own. She can better trust her own judgment when it is not being constantly attacked by her family.

Another major step. This meant trusting her ego. I was struck by how sane Elinor seemed in these comments. Where was her craziness? It was noteworthy that during the family sessions Elinor concluded that her parents would never change their views about sex and that she faced a therapeutic impasse. She simply could not stand the pressure their views placed upon her.

At the end of July in a family session Elinor's mother says that says Elinor has good news. She has been accepted by Penn's School of General Studies.

I noted that the mother was speaking for Elinor.

Throughout the session Elinor's eyes are downcast. I ask Elinor how she feels about this news. She says she thinks it will be difficult, but she will be able to handle it. She also thinks she's taking too much medicine. She has dizzy spells. I took her pulse and it was 100. She says her vision is blurred, her mouth dry, and she feels sleepy in the morning. I decrease her stelazine from 1 mg-3/d to 1/d.

In the next session she says she now feels confident to go her own way. She understands the family structure and how it operates and how she has fitted into it. She no longer feels prevented by family structure from developing her own nature. I say she will depend on friends. Elinor says she doesn't know how to meet friends.

After the session, Elinor's father says, "I already feel I've

lost a daughter. I don't want her back into the family the way she is. We are strangers! But I have to know what happened."

This sounded harsh. What was the matter with the way she was now? She seemed to be developing a mind of her own and be able to disagree with her father—which upset him. Why did he "have to know what happened?" This was part of defending his ego.

A September session after my vacation: Elinor's father says he no longer has a desire to understand Elinor's illness or his effect on Elinor if that means engaging in psychotherapy himself. Her mother says that she sees a steady growth in Elinor's self-confidence. The other day Elinor and Beth had a disagreement about whether the laundry required two washings or one. They turned to their mother for a decision. She said one load, though this meant siding with Beth. Elinor replied with flashing eyes that she still believed it required two washings and that they were both wrong!

She is most afraid of her grandmother, who says to her, "Why don't you just get with it!" Elinor suffers, too, from her grandmother's intrusive questioning. The grandmother would read both Elinor's and her mother's mail—and even her father's mail behind his back. Elinor's need for privacy is not honored by her grandmother or her mother—who always asks her father what he had for lunch. While Elinor was away at school and college, her mother expected her to write two or three times a week.

Elinor announces that the family sessions have been of enormous help, but now she wants to be on her own. Her parents agree to this and we all agree that no further family sessions will be scheduled. Her mother and father will contact me when they wish.

In mid-October the parents ask for a meeting. Her mother

says that Elinor told about making contact with an attractive young man who came and sat next to her. They reported, too, that she had asked her father if it was OK with him if she didn't get an "A." He replied indeed it was. It was an accomplishment just to get through the courses and that was enough for him. She also said she didn't want to return to college next semester. That, too, he could accept if it was her choice.

In November Doctor M. took a leave of absence and I began individual psychotherapy with Elinor.

In December she talks about the job she obtained as a store clerk. "It's been getting worse at work rather than better. I don't remember things. I keep asking questions, then can't remember the answers. I find myself apologizing to customers before they've asked me anything." I ask why she is working. She says, "I got backed into it by Doctor B. and my father."

She worked not because she wanted to but because she was "made to," an example of her deficient autonomy.

She continues, "It seems strange that I got A's at Princeton, but can't handle a clerk's job. I'm in bad shape today. My hands were trembling this morning at breakfast. My mother asked if I needed a sweater, and then she realized that wasn't the problem. I knew something was wrong with me, but didn't know it was fear until I got on the job. "I'm not sure what I'm afraid of. Maybe fear of being dumb."

She goes on, "I think I've become more immature since my illness. The pressure from my father always was that he'd think I'm dumb and the old pattern of asking questions and listening to his answers—which I've been using at work—no longer seems appropriate. It's too childlike. But I think I ought to be able to finish the nine days that are left. I want to prove something to myself."

This sounds more autonomous on her part, but her performance at work seems marginal. The stress is excessive. However, she seems motivated to continue. I raise her stelazine to 3 mg/day.

After seeing Elinor individually for X months, we had formed a therapeutic alliance and she had achieved considerable trust. Her relationships at home had arrived at a deeply negative impasse. She was again admitted voluntarily to the hospital.

Elinor says, "I never want to see my parents again."

The clinical sessions documented here took place during her first of ten years of treatment. After Elinor was discharged from the hospital, she lived by herself in an apartment for several years, retaining control and surviving on her own while seeing me as an out-patient. She began regularly raising her head and looking others in the eyes. She had her hair done in an attractive style. She wore skirts instead of jeans. She made this change to cause an effect that she wanted, namely to get a job. She had observed during job interviews that her unconventional costumes caused mistrust. She later married and lived with her husband in their own house and they had a daughter. She continued to see her parents frequently and with increasing harmony.

Though she was well on her way to resolving her conflict internally and with her family members, Elinor's struggles with her mother for autonomy lasted through much of the decade. In fact it was not until a second daughter had been born that Elinor had her breakthrough moment when "the worm turned" and she defied her mother for the first time in her life.

Her mother asked her to tend her parents garden and she refused. As she expected, her parents immediately cut off all relations.

Some days later she did agree to tend the garden because "It was nicer having them around." So Elinor had resolved her conflict between love and autonomy in favor of autonomy. Henceforth she could and would choose whether to comply or oppose a demand by her mother, or by any other person. No longer afraid, she was free to love and interact.

A few years after ending treatment, I received the following from Elinor, which I here excerpt:

Dear Doctor Appel,

In less than a month now, my daughter, Samantha, will be one year old—and what a delightful, amazing year it has been! Samantha is stupendous—curious, energetic, strong-willed, and demanding, with a devilish sense of humor and astounding blue eyes. She can crawl like the very Dickens and absolutely adores to have poor old mom (that's me) get down on her knees and chase her about. I rejoice to see her so lively and in such good health, because I know that means we've passed at least the first important hurdles successfully. Schizophrenia and motherhood are difficult enough to just think about in the same breath, let alone play them out in tandem on a day-to-day basis.

Building a life together with my husband Jim and Samantha makes me have to think about the various patterns and rituals that my parents adhered to with such self-righteous ferocity during the course of my childhood. My mother is generally ill-at-ease with Samantha, wanting her to come to her, rather than the other way around. . . . Observing how my mother reacts to Samantha's exuberant and mischievous spirit helps me understand a little better how I ended up as an adult feeling criminal and even dangerous.

I hope you are well. I still carry your voice in my head, and know I always will.

Chapter Six
Pathology of Autonomy — Dependence

People live by doing things. "To do is to be" means that if a person can't "do," he can't exist. To do things a person must be autonomous. A helpless person, dependent on others, will struggle for autonomy until he achieves it.

None of these three patients were autonomous. They were not able to choose what they did and so were unable to "be." They were helpless. Leslie was controlled by her rage and the "Lords." As she said, "I didn't do it, Emma did it . . . because the Lords told him to." Professor Marsh was controlled by his mother. As he said, "If you don't trust your own judgment you have to depend on someone else." Elinor was "crushed" by her father. He told her that what she thought was ridiculous." So she, too, was unable to "do" anything.

Domination threatens dissolution and loss of "self," nonexistence, the equivalent of death. It causes the greatest fear and rage experienced by humans. All three patients were angry, furious at their parents for controlling them. Leslie kept trying to strangle mother substitutes, banged her head and cut herself. She "shredded" people in her mind, peeling off their skulls, their brains, Professor Marsh could stand his mother's presence for only a few minutes because of his rage at her. Elinor kept her head down to hide murderous rage directed at her father.

The patients' rage represented their underlying unconscious

will to live, to exist, and so to take control of what they did— the drive for autonomy. The three patients were frightened, enraged, helpless, desperately lonely, in pain. These feelings were most intense while they were psychotic but were characteristic throughout their lives. Autonomy results in feeling pleased, strong, confident.

Although none of the three could control what they did, there was method in their madness—they could oppose control by others. Like a two-year-old they could say "no" and do the opposite of what they were told to do. Thus Leslie could and did refuse to eat, defecate, urinate, and cut herself, banged her head and tried to strangle older women, i.e., her mother—and refused to get well. Doing so gave her some sense of existing.

Professor Marsh refused to see his mother and finally, when he began to get well, refused openly to put on his overcoat when his mother told him to. Refusing relieved his pain, gave him some sense of existing.

Psychotic, Elinor could experience sexual feelings even though her parents told her sex was repulsive, and when she began to get well she defied her parents and acknowledged her sexuality openly, told them she hated them and never wanted to see them again. When, finally, for the first time in her life, she openly refused a request from her mother, both parents cut off all relationship with her. By that time she did not mind, because she had married and could get along without them.

These three patients were unable to oppose their parents openly while sane. They could do so only when "mad,"—had lost control of themselves and were not responsible for what they did. Recovery allowed them to oppose control by others deliberately and openly at last.

To oppose control by another person includes both: 1) refusing to do what that other one wants, and 2) freedom to do what one wants, even if doing so is opposed by the other person. Without autonomy a person finds himself doing things he doesn't want to do, but had been made to do by another person. And similarly, a dependent person is prevented from doing things he does want to do because another person doesn't want him to do them. He thus remains passive, unenterprising. To "control" a person means to make him do things he doesn't want to do and prevent him from doing things he does want to do.

Etiology

Autonomy develops ordinarily in childhood by interacting with a mother. The child finds he can do what he wants rather than what his mother wants. A mother who herself never went through the rebellion of the terrible twos, who lacks autonomy herself, cannot help her child attain it. If the mother could not oppose her own mother, she cannot tolerate her child saying "no" to her. To such a mother, the child's push for independence feels like an attempt to control her, dangerous, and is labeled "bad," "disobedient," and "selfish." She punishes the child's attempts with fierce scolding and withdrawal of love. She makes it clear to the child that if it persists it will lose her care. Two-year-olds cannot give up their mother, so they give up independence. They thus remain unable to do what *they* want; they become essentially timid, passive, submissive, without initiative, afraid to explore the world about them, or learn how to get along in it. To them their welfare is under their mother's control.

The conflict between autonomy and "love" continues until it is resolved, if ever, throughout a lifetime. How can a person resolve it? Only by gaining love from someone who accepts his autonomy. From a physician, at least, for starters.

What was the experience of the three patients in their terrible twos?

Leslie: Her mother "wished she'd never been born" and "didn't bring her up"; "tantrum over tooth brushing." Was her mother autonomous? Not likely.

Professor Marsh: A mother who "did not believe in viewpoints" would hardly permit her two-year-old child to have one.

Elinor: Raised by a controlling grandmother and a mother who cut her off when she refused a request.

So none of the three gained the power to choose what they did during the terrible twos, nor at any age until they found it in treatment. Their physician not only accepted their autonomy—he welcomed and even insisted on it.

Another patient, F., dependent, but not psychotic, at age seven refused to eat the food on her plate. Her mother pried open her mouth and thrust in food. Then, to force F. to swallow, her mother pinched F's nostrils and with the other hand covered F.'s mouth so she could not breath. F. vomited. Did F. refuse because she wasn't hungry? Or to take charge of her swallowing?

F. and her mother had been locked in a battle of wills since birth. In this moment she and her mother had a great deal at stake, nothing to do with nutrition. Each one thought she had to win. F. wanted control of her own life. It was her fight to establish an identity, to save her sanity.

The difference between an "adult" and a dependent person is possession of autonomous control. In command of what they think and do, adults no longer require the mother's permission for anything they do or think. Such autonomous people are even willing to give up the love of another person, rather than everlastingly submit to them. A dependent person is unable to contemplate such a choice. Being helpless, he would be lost without the care of the other on whom he depends. The consequences of not crossing the border into autonomous adulthood are significant and severe. Dependent people cannot attempt self-preservation, individuation and independence. They are too frightened to establish ego boundaries for themselves. They grow up inept socially and live in relative isolation because they are incapable of intimacy.

To survive and stay sane a person must have a repertoire of social behaviors. The three patients presented here were notably deficient socially. They were "weirdos," unable to respond to ordinary social cues, such as eye contact. Unable either to please others or maintain ego functions, they feared friendliness, feared domination and loss of ego. Psychiatric patients in general are poor at getting along with others. They make others uncomfortable; colloquially, they are variously boring, oversensitive, difficult, demanding, cold, pretentious, dominating, passive and notably poor spouses and parents, etc. However, they may be, as were the three patients, notably effective in non-social pursuits or professions.

Getting along with others is the most vital yet difficult thing a person must do to stay mentally well and survive. A person learns how to get along with people by getting along with his mother. He learns what pleases and what displeases her, and so learns how to be good or bad. He learns whether he may—or may not be autonomous—allowed by his mother to choose what he does. He thus gains a repertoire of behaviors. Normally these behaviors work pretty well with other persons. He modifies them, learning to get along with his father and siblings and later, other children. The person continues to use these patterns of behaviors as he grows into adulthood. They constitute his superego, his conscience and ideals internalized from his parents.

A person's superego represents parental authority internalized. The dynamics of a person's interaction with his conscience is similar to that of his interaction with his living external parents. And endless submission to his conscience can result in loss of identity just as so doing with his external parents. "Shoulds" can overwhelm a person and destroy him.

Dependent people have a different concept of justice than autonomous people. A dependent person expects to be treated the way his parents did and sees it as unfair to be punished for doing things they rewarded. They assume if they are fair to others, others will be fair to them. To not be rewarded is unfair; and to be punished for doing what is "right" more unfair. And then to witness someone else rewarded for doing something wrong is still more unfair, in fact, intolerable; it may depress them profoundly. However, parents may have had idiosyncratic, self-serving criteria of what is fair. There is no such thing as fairness; justice is a value judgment. An autonomous person is more apt to view it as such. He is more apt to judge fairness according to the consequences of what people do.

But whether patterns of behavior work and how well, depends on what the mother rewards. If she was absent, literally or because she was depressed and unresponsive, the child fails to develop any pattern of behavior—he remains irresponsible, a psychopath. Of course, a substitute mother can enable the child to develop to some extent, as can other family members. If the mother enjoyed her child, allowed the child to become autonomous, rewarded many of its behaviors, the behaviors work very well—other people reward them also.

Leslie said her parents didn't bring her up. She said her mother wished she'd never been born. Leslie's conscience was represented by the harsh White Lord, whose dictums were arbitrary, impossible to fulfill and demanded unquestioning total obedience. No autonomy was even remotely possible. Professor Marsh's conscience was equally severe, for example, demanding removal of his driver's license for any infringement of traffic regulations, no matter how trivial. Elinor's conscience was as sanctimonious as that of her father. So a person must become autonomous from his conscience as well as from his living parents. None of the three patients had become autonomous from either their parents or their superegos.

The struggle for autonomy was a key feature of the acute disabling psychosis in each patient. Also, all three patients had struggled for autonomy since childhood—a lifetime. Failure to achieve autonomy, and the resulting helplessness and dependence on their parents and their parents' rules led to their breakdowns. Leslie, for example, was twenty-three years old, a second year student in law school, when she cut her arm and showed it to her parents. Why did she have to resort to dramatic and violent means to get help? If she thought she needed to go to a doctor, why didn't she just go? She was unable to take such independent action; instead she turned to her parents to arrange it. Her father "liked to make decisions" for her. He decided she should go to law school and maintain the family tradition of achievement. If she did not want to got to law school, why did she go? Why didn't she go somewhere else? She was too uncertain and helpless. If everybody hated her so and she did not want to suffer the humiliation of social activities her mother chose for her, why did she attend them? Again, such independence was beyond her. For one thing she had not sufficiently differentiated from her mother to be clear about the difference between what she wanted and what her mother wanted.

Professor Marsh's mother made him put on an overcoat.

Why didn't he look at the thermometer and decide for himself whether to put it on? He was too helpless and dependent on his mother's opinion. And this was in spite of his eminence as a thinker in physics. He might know best about physics, but he thought she knew best about putting on overcoats. And he feared she might get mad at him if he disobeyed her. Then who would come and see him? Perhaps his woman friend, Felicia, would. But she would come two and one-half hours late and he'd have to wait; or she would want to borrow his car and he'd have to lend it to her.

Elinor screamed at her father, "You're so self-righteous! There I've said it," and buried her head in her mother's lap, sobbing quietly. Again, the point is her helplessness and dependence. Finally, after months of treatment, she dared oppose her father, in the safety of her mother's presence and mine. Why did it take her so long, why was it so dangerous? And why so important? Why did she mind his self-righteousness? She was unsure of her own opinion. If her opinion differed from her father's, and he was so sure he was right, then she concluded that she must be wrong. So she must abandon her opinion and accept his. But doing this undermined confidence in her ability to think at all. And if she could not trust her thinking how could she make decisions for herself, how could she direct her own life? He said what she thought was "ridiculous." Well, then, it must be so. Why even try to think for herself? Remain helpless and depend on him to think for her. But then she ceased to exist, she had no identity. If she opposed him he would cut her off. But she depended on him to take care of her. Her life, perhaps her sanity, depended on him. So she was caught both ways.

Psychosis represents loss of control, identity, autonomy, and desperate attempts to regain it.

In psychosis, psychic structure has broken down, with the resultant inability to perceive reality, or to evaluate the consequences of actions or indeed, the capacity to choose, decide to act. So Elinor sits frozen in her chair with her head down, Leslie and Professor Marsh sit glaring at the world. The three patients were in the equivalent of an experimental isolation tank, unable to affect their environment, but with no way out. Some individuals in an isolation tank retain their ego function by creating an imaginary environment, in which they do things, interact with other people, and have adventures. Leslie's "Kingdom" and "Lords" represented a similar use of fantasy to maintain her sense of existing.

In psychosis, both sensory and motor ego function are impaired: perceptions are distorted by various defenses: illusions, delusions, and projections. Leslie is unsure whether the "Lords" are inside her head or out. Professor Marsh perceives his world to be "upside down," and Elinor misperceives the men across the way in the next building to be looking at her, and "sees" the erections she arouses in them. She told me that when she entered a concert hall the conductor and the entire symphony orchestra immediately became aware of her presence and then performed for her personally. Leslie, who refers to herself as Emma, fears to act because her ego functions no longer control what she does; the "Lords," or her alter ego, Emma, take over, forcing her to strangle others or cut herself. Professor Marsh, when angered by the head nurse on his floor, imagines calling down the forces of Mars to destroy her and the entire world, including himself, in the process So he, too, must sit frozen and helpless.

The diagnosis "psychotic" has a cut-off point, and either/or quality. So does riding a bicycle or falling out of a window, or breathing. In the diagnostic category, "Borderline Personality," the "border" is between sanity and insanity. And the consequences of crossing the border are huge. The consequences of being a little "unhealthy" are not as obviously profound as being a little pregnant or losing balance while riding a bicycle. It might be argued that we all are a little psychotic, yet this is not true, we all are not dangerous to ourselves or others or need to be locked up. The cut off point is whether the person can or cannot survive independently, can or cannot perceive his environment realistically, or control what he does. The practical measurement of an individual's sanity and which side of the cut-off point the person is on is legally decided by a jury.

The jury uses the criterion of whether the person knows what he is doing and can control what he does. If so, the person is judged sane—he is held responsible and accountable. If not, he is adjudged insane and not guilty of the crime for which he is being tried.

Dependence

The pathology in psychosis has now been presented, illustrating the extreme helplessness involved with this disorder. What has not been presented is the pathology of lesser degrees of disability. Many people have not successfully navigated the terrible twos and so have remained dependent on others. But they nevertheless have managed to stay sane—have found a dependent way of living.

In psychosis, autonomy is almost entirely absent. Any or all ego functions are impaired to various degrees, but impaired sufficiently, by definition, to render the person helpless, unable to take care of himself and dangerous to others. Prior to the psychosis, though dependent, the patients did manage to stay sane —they adapted, coped with their circumstances adequately and at the same time maintained sanity. They had a degree of autonomy. Their ego functions, superego and physiologic drives did function adequately. Many people have not achieved full autonomy. They still depend on other people's decisions. They "get along by going along," although prone to mental disorder.

Any person may break down; every man has his breaking point. Whether or not he does break down depends on his vulnerability to stress and the circumstances he encounters. The three patients presented here did not encounter unusual stress. Yet Leslie broke encountering the ordinary responsibilities of adulthood, as did Elinor. Professor Marsh was able to cope as an adult, in fact, coped unusually well in his work, and actually survived military combat. He broke under stress which is ordinarily met successfully by most adults.

So the three patients broke down because, although adequate to that point in their lives, they lacked the competence to deal with ordinary circumstances they then encountered. Dependent people are vulnerable to stress normally tolerated by autonomous people. Their personality structure is defective. None of the three had achieved psychological adulthood, none had become autonomous, able to function independently. They had survived by depending on decisions provided them by their parents, or by their internalized parents—superegos, ideals and consciences.

For these children, afraid to oppose anyone, offers of love, of friendships, or of any kind of interaction becomes dangerous, a threat to identity and sanity. Yet a person needs interaction in order to survive. Dependent children keep on struggling to gain autonomy throughout their lives. But they remain babies—a mama's boy or girl—submitting to mama's decisions rather than their own. Severely limited in their interactions, they are timid and passive—and their submission and compliance brings them some sense of security. But they continue to rage, often unconsciously, at their impotence. They are prone to mental disorder.

While doing things is the principle way to gain autonomy, refusing is another way. Some children during "the terrible twos" do develop a degree of autonomy. But this is only a half rebellion. The mother, by making the demand, is backhandedly determining the outcome. The child, when doing the opposite, is still controlled. The only true liberating independence is choice—the ability to say yes or no without reference to the mother's wishes.

Autonomy incurs responsibility for the consequences of actions and gives the person a sense of existing. An autonomous person seeks and accepts this responsibility. He assumes he is responsible for his existence and well-being. A dependent person, although sane, assumes other people are responsible for him. Like the patient, J, who believed her husband was responsible for her pain and unhappiness, not realizing she was responsible and should have opposed his control.

A dependent person will go to almost any length to avoid responsibility. Every morning at home a patient named Mrs. B. asked her five children, plus her husband, what each wanted for breakfast. She cooked and served six different menus, not including her own. This extended to asking each child how he wanted his toast: light, medium, or dark brown. And if a child changed his mind on seeing his brother's toast, she redid a slice. Doing all this and getting the children off to school on time made mornings a horrible experience.

This helps explain why Mrs. B became psychotic every few months and had to be hospitalized. To prepare and serve a single menu for breakfast was beyond her. She could not risk the annoyance of her children. She could not evaluate the consequences of her actions and take the responsibility of refusing any demand, so she assigned responsibility to everyone. Anything wrong would be their fault, not hers.

A woman patient, Professor R., was told she must always put her parents first. She was told that it was unacceptable, a crime, to get herself a glass of water without first offering one to each parent. In treatment she once said, "to do what I want is an impossible dream. All I can think of is how to do what the other person wants."

A child's drive for self-preservation by putting its needs first is deemed "selfish" by many parents and punished severely—and consequently is prohibited by the patient's conscience. "Being good" is made to matter more than finding out how to get along in the world, is made to be the way to get along. As a result, people may be confident about what is right and wrong, but highly unsure about their judgment of consequences, of cause and effect.

In our culture avoiding responsibility has a glossary of semantic devices: "Look what you made me do." "It would be nice if you. . . ." A mother says to her child, "You don't want more candy," and thereby avoids both the responsibility and blame for refusing to dispense it. She does not risk the child's anger and the feeling that maybe she is a mean, bad mother. The child who says, "I do so want more candy" doubts the validity of his perceptions. The confusion affects the value he places on his feelings.

Dependent people do not think of the effect of what they do, particularly the effect on others. They may do a wide range of things on their own. But they are not truly independent. They assume their parents or others are responsible for consequences of such acts. Anything they do is still, in effect, under parental control.

Lacking a clear concept of cause and effect, of responsibility, they tend to bond with another dependent person. In such interdependent relationships, each is offering to take care of and submit to the other person. Using the power of helplessness is the chief way that dependent people secure the care they need.

This sets up circular love: "I'll do what you say and you will do what I say." "I'll take care of you and you will take care of me." "I'll love you because you love me." Such love has relatively little to do with the actual characteristics of either individual. It neither threatens, nor rewards them. Perhaps surprisingly, such relationships may endure for a lifetime.

In such marriages each bickers constantly with the other over trivial issues. "But you said you'd be home by 6:00!" "No dear, I said I'd try to be home by 6:30." "I distinctly remember you said 6:00." "No, I said 6:30." The real issue is not time, but who is right and who is wrong—and identity confusion. The closer the bond, the greater the need to keep identities distinct. Autonomous partners can more easily think, "Well, we have different opinions about the time."

Similar identity problems occur to some degree in most people in most relationships. However, the issue is not simply the ability to say a flat "no" to a command or demand. People develop various categories of response. For example, lovers, particularly somewhat dependent ones, may seek clues to the slightest wish of the beloved and then go to any lengths to fulfill it. Saying "no" to the beloved's wish is just as unthinkable as refusing a direct demand—"If you love me you will do what I say." Or people may easily say "no" to strangers but not to loved ones. Or else they can say "no" to a command, but not to a request, particularly a plea for help.

Agnes, a fifty-four-year-old patient afraid of opposing anyone, hated answering the telephone. If her best friend, Mabel, was calling, she would have to stay on the phone as long as two and one-half hours listening to her friend's troubles. She was helpless to end the call. I asked her why she couldn't just tell her friend she had to stop. "Oh, I couldn't do that," she replied. "Mabel would get mad at me."

Fearful as she was of the phone, Agnes once stayed home all day waiting for a call from her sister. I asked why. She said, "Well, sister said she might call and she'd be mad if I wasn't there." Every few months Agnes became psychotic, suicidal, and had to be kept in the ward for violent patients. Once, in her rage, she suddenly ran from the isolation room where we were talking and locked me in.

People like Agnes depend on the opinion of others for their opinion of themselves, and are unable to judge for themselves who or what they are. They place themselves under the control of anyone with whom they interact, answer any questions, permit any intrusion, accept any insult, believe any criticism, take the role of the defenseless, willing victim. As such victims, they then forbid themselves to fight or flee, or even to defend themselves, let alone counterattack. Dependent people mistrust their own judgment and follow the judgments of others. Doing so leaves them helpless, at the mercy of the opinions of other people.

This is particularly dangerous when dependent people judge themselves. They believe any insult, any accusation of blame. They are unable to think, "Well, that's his opinion," and make an independent evaluation of their behavior which may or may not be in agreement. And they are vulnerable to sycophancy, unable to assess praise. To them any disagreement presents a crisis. They must either prove the other wrong or give up their own opinion. They are unable to just disagree and not have to straighten out the other person.

Such automatic and obligatory submission to control by others is a way of making the other person decide. It bypasses ego function—which forfeits identity. Such helpless people remain ignorant of their environment and how to affect it. They remain malfunctioning and vulnerable to mental disorder.

Dependent people still need a mother's control and panic if left on their own. To function as adults, they need this mythical, loving, good person who cares for them. Knowing that they would be lost without a mother, they get a stand-in to look after them, to do everything from making most decisions to balancing their checkbook.

Anger in a child frequently, if not always, is deemed "bad" by parents, particularly when directed at the mother. Yet the anger is part of the energy for the fight-flight reflex necessary for survival and for sanity. When a mother prohibits other such basic drives, the result may be a conflict that can lead to psychopathology. A common arena of autonomy struggle is eating, a collision with parents for control of what and how much the child eats can lead to anorexia nervosa, bulemia, obesity, and substance abuse. Similar conflicts occur at the potty.

Having to be right—like F.'s mother, like the patient Elinor's father—is a heavy burden

Chapter Seven
Taking Charge

"A person does, or tries to do what makes him feel good" is almost a truism, variously seen as axiomatic, or as immoral; viz. people should do what makes others feel good, not themselves. Of course, a person can claim it makes him feel good to make others feel good, but this claim in turn can be challenged: a truly moral person tries to make others feel good, even if doing so make him feel bad. Pursuit of self-interest in any guise may be deemed selfish or bad. However, self-preservation can be distinguished from selfishness, and seen as good, a responsibility of an individual.

What does make a person feel good? The man on the street would like to know. The question is fundamental to a physician. Knowing the answer to this question is his professional responsibility, his means of earning his living. Patients feel bad—they feel pain. The physician is supposed to relieve their pain. Mental disorder is painful, patients feel bad. The psychiatrist is supposed to relieve their pain. So how does a physician relieve pain?

The answer, for the man on the street as well for the physician, may be sought psychologically or physiologically. The physiological answer is primary for physicians of all types. A surgeon can cut out the tumor, for example, which causes the pain, or set the broken bone. The issue differs when treating patients with mental disorders, in whom the cause of pain may not be primarily physiological. Sigmund Freud claimed man is governed by "the pleasure principle." And it is astonishing how many words in the English language denoting motives are partners in dichotomies activated by pleasure, or displeasure. For example: success/pleasure vs. failure/pain; love/pleasure vs. hate/pain; hunger/pain vs. eating/pleasure; etc. So then feeling good means gaining pleasure and avoiding pain. And indeed, Epicurus, two thousand years ago, said pleasure and pain are the two feelings by which choice and avoidance are determined.

The answer—the way to feel good is to seek pleasure and avoid pain. Is such a notion simplistic? Simplistic or not, is it true? And what is pleasure? Can it be observed? Measured? Pleasure is repeated.

How then does a person gain pleasure? "Do unto others as you would have others do unto you," is one answer. "Be of service," is another. These answers are not of much help to a physician, a psychiatrist, or other specialist. Treating psychotic patients does suggest an answer. To reward a psychotic patient's behavior when interacting with him makes him feel good.

Drugs are, of course, a help. Some psychiatrists believe only drugs are effective. However, rewarding psychotic patients' behavior in therapeutic interaction seems to make them feel good. In fact, doing so, along with other psychological measures and with drugs, cures them.

Seeking and gaining rewarding responses when interacting with others not only cures psychiatric patients, but makes the man on the street feel good.

How does a physician help an assaultive, suicidal, self-cutting patient like Leslie? Or a professor who bursts into a University President's office, and says he's upside down and is communicating by brain waves? Or a young woman who hides in her room because she "sees" men's erections, aroused by the heat of her body. The first thing the physician does is take control of the patients' behavior, in a locked hospital if necessary.

For months Leslie was tied hand and foot. But her ego, her identity, the inner "me" was not at stake. Her identity was not in her muscles, but in her brain—her ego. Her physician controlled her muscles, not her ego. He took great care to avoid any attempt to control her thoughts or decisions. He never told her to stop banging or cutting, for example. Leslie welcomed such control by her physician. In full physical restraints, she said "It feels so good to fight as hard as I want, yet know I can't hurt myself or anyone else." The physician rewarded her head-banging by having nurses go to her and hold her physically—bodyguards who concurrently gave her comfort. Self-destructiveness could be abandoned when she found more constructive ways of interacting.

The goal of the patient and the physician is to replace such external control with internal control, accomplished by rewarding ego function—internal control. Just as a mother rewards her child's behavior, the physician rewards his patient's behavior. No matter how helpless he is, a patient seeks human interaction to relieve his desperate loneliness. The physician recognizes the patient's efforts and rewards them.

The physician's early task is to diagnose his patients' techniques of interacting—which are markedly deficient and a major reason for psychosis. But patients must use the limited techniques they already possess. Desperate for interaction, they attempt to elicit responses from the physician. The physician must reward these behaviors, even though deficient, in order to keep the patient alive. He must continue to do so throughout treatment until the patient has developed new, effective behaviors and other persons with whom to interact.

The physician becomes like a mother who rewards and penalizes her dependent child—but this mother has different criteria for "good" and "bad," chooses different issues for opposition. This mother is autonomous, is not threatened by disagreement or disobedience. This mother, giving pleasure or pain, renders his patient's actions successful or unsuccessful, thereby nurturing an ability to interact. And the patient develops new adaptive behaviors.

The patient does things: weeps, complains, bangs her head, boasts, and smiles at the physician. He, or she, tells dreams, analyzes his behavior, tells his motives. The physician, responding, rewards the patient by expressing sympathy to the weeping, listens to the complaints, interprets the dreams, When the patient seeks agreement, or validation of his opinion, the physician provides it, if he thinks it warranted; if the patient seeks understanding of his behavior or motives, the physician gives his suggestions. He negatively rewards unadaptive behaviors, such as refusing to eat. He thus strengthens the patient's repertoire. Such strengthening represents strengthening ego-autonomy. He serves as a surrogate mother, but rewards different behavior than did the patient's real mother.

When patients say things, the physician responds by listening and responding. No matter what the physician says, the very fact he responds makes the patient's action successful. The patient does not feel helpless. If the physician's response is what the patient wanted, the pleasure is even greater. Standard theory might require the physician to not reply to the patient's question, except, perhaps to inquire, or suggest why the patient asked the question. This nonresponse leaves the patient helpless and discouraged.

The physician proceeds on the assumption that patients' words and behaviors do have an adaptive intent. His competence is to discern the patient's underlying intent and respond to it. For example, the physician assumed Leslie banged her head to gain attention and to prove her independence. He responded accordingly, having the nurses pay attention to her and and hold her. The physician's presumption of validity communicates itself to patients and validates their ego functions.

There is the argument that such reward will, in fact, foster dependence and make patients worse. This is not supported by clinical observation. Every human has a powerful innate urge to be in control of himself. Just as the infant seizes the spoon and tries to feed itself, so all patients constantly seek to direct their own behavior. Rewarding these attempts reinforces them.

As biological organisms, normal human beings survive by learning to interact with their environment. People remember and repeat rewarded behavior and avoid what has failed or been punished. They develop a repertoire of adaptive behaviors, knowing which will please and attract, or oppose and repel.

The brain has an extensive reward system[39]. It extends as a dopaminergic projection from the hind brain, up through the mid-brain and well into the frontal lobes of the fore-brain. This reward system controls the organism's adaptive interaction with the environment, including the social environment.

In treatment, the patient does something, asks the physician a question, for example, the psychological equivalent to pressing a lever. The physician answers the patient's question. The lever was wired to the rat's brain. Instead of going by wire, the physician's answer goes as sound waves to the patient's ear and thence to his brain reward system . Gaining reward from asking a question impels the patient to repeat the act, "press the lever" again, e.g., ask another question. This act is rewarded. The patient remembers question-asking brings pleasure and so this behavior is "strengthened." Similarly, other behaviors are rewarded and so reinforced by the physician.

Interaction between patient and physician is a vastly complicated process, involving even as many a thousand transactions per minute, as shown by Birdwhistle[40]. Facial expressions, tones of voice, postural movements—all nonverbal as well as verbal communications—may reward or not reward the patient or the physician. Familiar elements of interaction such as friendliness and hostility, warmth and coolness, are transmitted by a vast, exquisitely nuanced repertory of visual, auditory, tactile and other physical elements: the visual clues in facial expressions.

Learning how to interact involves change in the patient's personality structure, including self-object representation, parental representation, super-ego formation, and their dynamic interplay. This change requires release of developmental arrests and resumption of growth so that deficits are removed. Resolution of basic conflicts between autonomy and the need for nurturance is necessary but in itself an insufficient element in the process.

The patient's conscience represents the mother's rules of behavior, internalized. Treatment is to enable the patient to become adult in this respect, autonomous from the mother and her rules. If the internalized superego rules are maladaptive, then the therapeutic task is not only to gain autonomy from them, but to change them. Or if the rules are absent and insufficient due to parental absence or neglect, the task is to develop new codes of behavior. Patients project their code of behavior—their vision of right and wrong—onto the physician. During their interaction, they begin to perceive, consciously and unconsciously, that the physician's code differs from theirs, that he rewards behavior differently than did the patient's mother or her rules. They come to adopt elements of that code. Thus, the goal of treatment is not to replace or dispense with the superego, but to develop one based on ego function which is used as a guide, rather than an authority for social interaction. The patient gains a new concept of justice based on cause and effect. For example, Professor R. was surprised to realize that if she failed to arrange a meeting with a companion she "deserved" to be lonely, it was her fault.

Locked into a lifelong pattern of doing what other people want, patients are astounded when rewarded for doing what they want, rather than what the physician wants—or more specifically, what patients think the physician wants. Leslie found it "unbelievable" that her physician would listen to—reward—her when she talked about what she wanted. The same with Elinor, especially when her physician did not find her thoughts "ridiculous." The countless interactions with the physician, minute by minute, rewarding and validating, overcome the weakening effect of parental derogation.

Initially, patients feel helpless in the face of the physician's immense power. Then they begin to realize that, in fact, they themselves have the ability and power to affect the physician's behavior. Causing him to laugh, look sad, frightened, angry, gives them a sense of power. In causing him to be affectionate, respectful, delighted, they experience control, the physician becomes a source of self-esteem, of attention and companionship, of practice in evoking the same reactions in others—the means to survive and stay sane.

The patients are discovering that they can reward or oppose the physician. Furthermore, they realize that it is not their duty to please the physician. It is his job to reward them. For many patients this power is almost incomprehensible and only gained step by step. They may have to test the physician repeatedly to prove it to themselves.

As in the "terrible twos," patients test the mother/physician from opposite directions. Can they say no to him? Can he say no to them? As the answers become "yes," they are learning separation and self-direction, learning that they can make choices with the mother/physician—and therefore with anybody else.

More importantly, they learn they cannot say "yes" if they cannot say "no"—and cannot say "no" if they cannot *accept* "no."

For dependent people, any dispute endangers their credibility and therefore sanity. So they are unable to collaborate, unable to believe anything unless another person agrees. When Leslie advanced her idea that her parents had not brought her up, the physician validated her opinion. He showed interest and rewarded her as she elaborated. The physician, being autonomous, was free to decide what response he would make, free to judge whether her behavior was adaptive and, accordingly, whether to reward or oppose her. If there was a disagreement, he did not have to change her opinion or give up his own. This freedom communicated itself to Leslie and allowed her to talk freely to him.

Patients see that the physician does not require agreement or compliance. In fact, he welcomes independent thinking in his patients—it is the goal of treatment. He wants their opinions to change, but only on the basis of their own judgment. Thus patients are escorted in treatment through the terrible twos that they never dared experience in their childhood.

A patient's progress is sometimes tracked in dreams. Frequently it is represented by driving an automobile. For example, a patient named James dreamed that he was a passenger in his father's car. This meant his father, not James, was running his life. Later he dreamed he was in his own car, but his father was at the wheel. Here James was protesting that his father was not going where James wanted to go. This dream showed progress in achieving autonomy. His life was his own and he could protest, even if his father was still at the controls. Still later in treatment James dreamed that he was riding a bicycle by himself along a narrow mountain ledge. Here at last he had taken over from his father and was running his own life—even though autonomy—the mountain ledge—seemed extremely dangerous.

During successful treatment there comes a moment of new maturity. The worm turns. The patient turns from helplessness to power—the power to interact with anybody. The patient openly and directly declines to answer a question asked by the physician. Leslie was able to say "I did it," not her alter ego, Emma, not The Lords. Professor Marsh disobeyed a direct order from his mother to put on his overcoat. Elinor told her father he was sanctimonious, and said, "no," to a request from her mother.

Central to a patient's discovery of control is the realization that independence—the power to decide—is internal. While people must depend on others for survival, it does not follow that they must depend on others for *decisions*. They have the power to choose whether to comply with any demand, or whether to acquiesce sufficiently to maintain a relationship with a particular person. Ordinarily, this realization takes place during the "terrible twos"[38, 20].

The physician must never undermine his patient's trust by seeking to get the patient to benefit *him* in some way. He should respond to patients with interest, sympathy, understanding, admiration, and affection when the patient does things intended to obtain these responses—provided the physician can do so honestly. If the patient tells a joke—and *if* it strikes the physician—he should laugh, rewarding the patient. But the physician should not tell jokes to seek pleasure from the patient's laughter.

The fact that the physician is paid a fee liberates him from any responsibility to act in his own interests and forbids him from seeking responses for his own benefit. Money is his reward, not his own ego enhancement.

The effect of failing to abide by this principle is illustrated by the catastrophic case reported by Peter Knapp[45] in 1983. He was treating a young woman for psychogenic asthma attacks and she was showing steady progress. Then suddenly in the middle of a session she developed status asthmaticus which failed to respond to emergency treatment and she died in the office. Afterward, reviewing his notes of the session, Doctor Knapp realized that just before the asthma attack, he had asked her a question designed to serve his research interests rather than to benefit her. After a lifetime of exploitation by her mother, his question betrayed her developing trust that he would be different, that he would devote himself to her interests. Her resultant rage and despair precipitated the status asthmaticus which killed her.

The principle that the physician must never take advantage of patients in any way does pose a paradoxical inconsistency. Even as he must always act for their advantage, he must also be ready to act for his own interests by physically protecting himself. When assaulted by Leslie, her physician left the room and locked the door behind him. He did not do so for her benefit, but for his own.

However, such an incident can help patients. The next day, Leslie told her physician that she was so glad he had escaped and locked the door. Patients fear the damage that their rage, their uncontrolled behavior, might do. They are immensely reassured to find that the physician can and does defend himself. Moreover, he becomes a model, showing vulnerable patients how to defend themselves.

An important exception to the rule of self-benefit concerns the physician's fee and his time. Patients are responsible for the fee. Here the physician should interact in his own interests and do what is necessary to induce the patient or his representatives to pay. If patients dispute the fee, symbolic issues may be involved: "caring" for the patient, "liking" him, power, respect etc. Therefore, it is therapeutically useful to analyze such disputes. But in resolving the dispute, the physician must interact for his benefit. Otherwise, the physician invalidates his relationship with the patient.

Particularly, in the beginning of each session, a key element is who chooses the topics or the transactions. A therapeutic assumption is that patients always have something they want to talk about, or something they want to get from the physician—attention at least, or validation, or sympathy. But patients dare not seek what they want. They attempt to do what they think the physician wants, try to make him choose the topic. He opposes such requests or demands. A battle of wills is frequent.

The task of the physician is to ascertain his patients' underlying wants and try to meet them. But patients develop ego capacity from what they do, not what the physician does—primarily facilitating and rewarding. By analogy, the professional positions the tennis ball for the learner to hit. Patients have a tendency to reverse the role and position balls for the professional to hit. This is their dependent style of trying to please the other person.

An example of pathologic helplessness and compliance treated by interaction is a patient named Mr. M. He said, "The reason you like me is because I do what you want me to do." He explained, "If you ask me a question I must answer it, or try to, and I feel guilty if I fail. Or when you say something I have to listen and agree. I have to suspend my own judgment because it might lead to disagreement, and you would stop liking me and end our relationship." He continued, "I am helpless in any close relationship. So I keep others at a distance. I have no idea what intimacy is. I can't conceive of being able to disagree in a relationship." Treating Mr. M. required showing him that he could disagree with me and I would continue to like him.

The physician does use conventional psychoanalytic techniques: free association, dream analysis, interpretations, etc. The primary aim in conventional psychoanalytic treatment has been to bring unconscious defenses and motives into awareness. However, this has limited value in treating psychotic patients. The limitations of interpretations as a means of therapeutic change have now been recognized by many writers, but more effective means have yet eluded them.

In treating psychosis, the primary aim is to reward adaptive behavior. The psychotic patient's behavior is maladaptive, and cannot be made adaptive solely through the physician providing insight. It is noteworthy that developing insight is not normally part of child rearing. The physician focuses on ego functions, because that is where the chief pathology lies. Unable to interact effectively, patients are unable to anticipate the effects of their actions, and misperceive the behavior of others. They do not know how to please or oppose others. This ego pathology is rooted in ignorance and mistaken ideas of how to interact with other people. It is not just the result of repressed unconscious object representations or affects. The process of adopting new ways and discarding old ones may require overcoming resistance due to repression, but much of a patient's response is acquiring concepts that are new and not resisted by him.

The physician's "interpretations," "interventions," "confrontations," etc., are social interactions—just one type among the myriad that constitute therapy. Therapeutic interaction is merely a type of social interaction and is composed of all the elements of any social interaction. The patient and analyst constantly do things to affect each other, to elicit responses from each other. Though conscious insights are a vital element of treatment, it is not the insights that the physician provides which cure, but the physician's affective, cognitive, verbal, non-verbal responses—his laughter, sympathy, irritation, attention, and understanding.

A smile by the physician may have more therapeutic power than any interpretation. A smile is a part of an interaction between the entire personalities of both participants. This is not to say interpretations do not have therapeutic value—but not until patients have become strong enough to use the knowledge gained to cause a smile, frown, or other response which makes them feel good.

An interpretation by the physician can please patients interpersonally in addition to revealing unconscious dynamics. They feel rewarded by a sense that the physician understands them, by a feeling that they now have a new promise of mastery, of being in charge; a sensation of autonomy! What could be more gratifying or rewarding than to be truly listened to for fifty minutes a day for months or years? Most people have difficulty getting anyone to listen for more than a few minutes, let alone finding a person who responds to them with comprehension. This, indeed, is an "ego trip."

When psychotic patients deliberately try to annoy, a reaction of annoyance from the physician reinforces adaptive behavior. Yet success of treatment depends on the physician liking and respecting his patients, on his ability to gain satisfaction from interacting with his patient, even though psychotics are unattractive, unlikable, expert at making others uncomfortable.

The limited terms of the therapeutic relationship makes the physician's continued liking of them possible. Since the physician does not need to have patients enjoy him and boost his self-esteem, he does not set himself up to be hurt. He does not make advances which can be snubbed. He does not show off, and try to impress with his professional skill or social virtues.

The physician can be pleased by things the patients choose to do. If nothing they do pleases him, he cannot reward them, cannot treat them. But he must show genuine pleasure. Insincerity, feigned pleasure, is immediately detected and rejected by the patient. Sometimes honest demonstrations of liking may be misinterpreted. A major element of pathology is incredulity and consequent misreading of signs that the other person honestly cares.

Thus, the physician treats patients with his feelings as well as with his thoughts and knowledge. A degree of "caring" joins the panorama of human emotions he shares—along with anger, fear, competitiveness, affection, love, and even an appropriate degree of sexual feelings.

This chapter dealt with treatment of psychoses—extreme mental disorders. The means used for this purpose are also effective treating less severe disorders: neuroses, addictions, personality disorders. The same means are also useful to normal people when interacting with others in their daily lives—particularly when resolving conflicts of intent or opinion.They can be used at work, in school, in politics, and in law.

Chapter Eight
Staying Sane: Autonomous Living

An autonomous person wakes up in the morning and thinks, what do I want to do today? Then he gets out of bed and does it, or at least tries to: goes to work, wakes up the children, prepares a lecture for tomorrow's class. Many of the things he decides to do are things he should do anyway. He deals with the stresses of the day.

Psychotic patients have broken down from normal stress. Genetic "weakness" is not necessary to explain their vulnerability. They have been rendered vulnerable by phenomena sadly common—by parents who dominated them, who didn't "listen" and dismissed their thought processes. One patient, Leslie, broke when she went to school and failed to make friends. She thought everybody hated her. Another, Elinor, broke trying to cope with boyfriends. Well, you probably have your own doubts about whether people like you. Elinor thought everyone noticed her sexual arousal. Well, have you ever worried that people noticed when your skirt was too tight?

When another patient, Professor Marsh, broke, he was failing at work where he could not cope with rebellious subordinates, and he was isolated, with "no one to talk to." He felt compelled to comply when his mother told him to put on his overcoat. Well, you may find it hard to resist when your wife tells you, "That necktie doesn't match. Put on another one." And does this sound familiar? "My glasses, where are my glasses? I had them a minute ago, I must be going out of my mind."

You are probably thinking "OK, I have some of those same problems, but, my God, I am not about to go crazy." True, of course. One patient never had any friends. You, at least, have someone to talk to. Obeying his mother made Professor Marsh so angry he had to leave the room. You probably don't do everything your wife says. Unlike Leslie, when you get mad at your wife, you do not actually try to strangle her. And if you are a woman, unlike Elinor, you do not "see" men having erections in response to your short skirt. And you do finally find your glasses. There they are, right under your nose.

The possibility that anybody can break down mentally may be terrifying. You may be eager to deny it. Even so, your next, perhaps urgent, question might be, "What can I do to stay sane?"

The first step is to do something. Act. Cause something to happen. Especially do something that elicits a response from another person. "Well," you say, "I am constantly doing things. I'm busy, perhaps too busy, at work and trying to raise a family, trying to do good."

"Fine," I reply. "There are plenty of reasons to do these things, but you probably don't realize that these activities are what keep you sane." When you do whatever makes you feel good, this is the same method a psychotic patient uses in treatment to get well. Leslie and Professor Marsh sought reward and obtained it by talking to their physician. Leslie said that being listened to was the most wonderful thing that had happened in her life.

The concept of pleasure/reward and pain/punishment explains many areas of behavior. Your brain has a reward system and you remember what was rewarded and what was punished.

You repeat the former and avoid the latter. Furthermore, you must decide for yourself what you do. Submitting to the decisions of others does not help your mental health, and may actually harm it. Of course you have to do what your boss tells you. But not just because he tells you. You always have a choice.

This means that you must take responsibility for what you do—take credit and risk blame—or remain forever helpless. Like Leslie when "the worm turned," you must be able to say, "I did it!" without refuge in blaming others—Leslie's claim that "Emma did it." So it is what you do that keeps you sane, not what someone else does.

Unfortunately, autonomy often conflicts with what someone else wants you to do. Getting along with people is the chief source of both your pleasure and pain in life—and the vital necessity for your sanity. But your most difficult challenge is attracting others while defending yourself from being dominated by them.

Like most people you may not be altogether confident in your ability to do either successfully. You use the same methods you developed during the "terrible twos" for getting along with your parents and siblings. These strategies may work very well with the people in your present life, or they may not.

But like Professor Marsh, you must have someone who will listen while you talk. Just as you must breathe to stay alive, you must interact to stay sane. In that isolation tank you would float in an environment that you could not affect. But some people, by conjuring a flow of imagination, do manage to stay sane by interacting with themselves. Most people do not return to their senses until they emerge and resume normal interactions.

As mentioned above, being active in nonsocial activities also, to a limited extent, enables you to stay sane. For example, Leslie helped her mental health considerably by teaching herself Greek. Professor Marsh's improvement took a big jump when he could resume physics. But things do not actively respond to what you do. People react.

In any relationship one intuitively tests the autonomy of the other and adjusts accordingly. For example, you test whether others compulsively need to be always right. Or can they listen to what you say with an open mind? Such freedom is sought by everybody. Like Professor Marsh, you hate being controlled, told what to think and do. You hate constantly giving in. But you may not recognize the reason that this reaction is so strong. Your mental health is involved. You are defending your sanity.

Now let's get down to the nitty-gritty. Saying no to a loved one, that's the hard part. The choice whether to oppose or comply comes up constantly in relationships, often over apparently trivial matters. If you give in too often, there will be no more you left, no more identity. But if the issue between you and your wife is important, and you say no to her, can you stand the reaction? Maybe the silent treatment. Maybe even tears? Or in the extreme: When Elinor, for the first time in her life said no, her parents cut off all relations with her.

So power in a relationship is the willingness to make this choice, the willingness to risk a person's love. You cannot "have" someone unless you are willing to give them up. This sounds like a terrifying brinkmanship. It feels next to impossible to replace a loved one, particularly a person as important as your mother or spouse. But to get well, each of those three patients had to find the courage to risk saying no to their parents and to anyone else, while attracting replacements—friends and others willing to interact.

In marriage, conflicts arise minute by minute—whether to

have cereal for breakfast, how to discipline a child, and so on. How then does one resolve conflicts without losing either love or sanity? You collaborate. If you and the other person are grownups, able to disagree with each other without panicking, without having to win—you can find a resolution acceptable to both. Not all conflicts are autonomy conflicts. In the case of TV, for instance, you can bargain for programs, gaining equal access to your choice. It helps for each to give the other veto power over any proposed solution, then each of you can relax, knowing you cannot be controlled by the other. The same principles apply to being right. You can resolve disagreements of opinion if you can admit you are wrong without losing your dignity—or sanity.

Resolution of conflicts becomes more complicated if neither of you is adult and both dependent. In that case collaboration is impossible. Conflicts then must be resolved by one or the other giving in. One solution, common in marriages, is assigning separate domains of authority: the wife has the say indoors, the husband outdoors, etc. But, of course, conflicts and their resolution are not confined to marriage. They occur in all relationships. And, designation of domains is not possible in many instances, for example, in friendship.

But bear in mind that powerful, bossy people are in fact not powerful at all, rather the opposite. Like Mrs. Goldman, they are usually childlike, dependent, weak, desperately trying to control everyone to preserve their own identity.

When one of you is autonomous, the other dependent, you can resolve conflicts somewhat more easily. The autonomous one can give in frequently for the sake of harmony, reserving "no" only for issues which seem vital—usually money or welfare of children.

Doing what you want to do—though often considered self-indulgent and selfish—is vital to your sanity. But this autonomy requires that you take into account the consequences of your wants. You may modify your "want" because you fear alienating a close friend. You may want to punch someone in the nose, but after considering that the other may punch you back, you may change your mind. As an adult you can prevent your feelings from controlling you.

Conversely, realize that you may be angry without knowing it, or frightened, or unaware that you are making sexual advances. You, like everyone, are profoundly influenced by motives and beliefs buried in your so-called "unconscious." For example, you may hold "choice" in abortion as a cause to live or die for—quite unaware that your passion comes from experience with your mother, who never allowed you to choose anything. Similarly, your passionate insistence on privacy may come from your lack of it as a child. Your basic expectations of getting rewards from others may come from your success—or failure—as a child trying to please your mother. Knowing that all people are full of unconscious prejudices, rationalizations and biases may enable you tolerate irrationalities in others—and in yourself.

You may take for granted that being nice, being considerate of others, putting the other fellow first, is the way to go. And, of course, it is. However, keep in mind that doing so beyond a certain point can destroy your identity. Your first responsibility is to stay sane, even if doing so entails putting self-interest ahead of pleasing some one else. Selfishness differs from self-preservation.

Similarly, you assume that doing what you "should" do is good. It is the basis of civilization. But remember that doing it to excess can drive you insane. You can be overwhelmed by shoulds. So in any particular instance you must consider the consequences and make a calculated decision. In every situation, there is always a choice, perhaps not a good one, but a choice.

So sanity includes autonomy not only from demands of other people and from "shoulds," but also from compelling emotions: temper, fear, lust, greed. You cannot control whether you have these feelings, only what you do about them.

Measurable* Signs of Mental Health

You:
- — Can tell, roughly, what day it is, what your name is and where you are.
- — Are active, intentionally causing effects by interacting with your surroundings.
- — Are autonomous: deciding for yourself what you do.
- — Recognize and use customary social cues, such as greetings and eye-contact.
- — Predict, roughly, the effect of what you do, particularly the effect on other people.
- — Know how to reward and get reward from other people.
- — Initiate activities.
- — Attract others and yet can say no to their demands.
- — Acknowledge the existence of your biases and unconscious motivations.
- — Manage your money.
- — Have someone who is almost always glad to see you and will come to your funeral.

* It can be argued that mental health cannot be measured because it is subjective, not objective. Particularly, that the intent or goal of behavior is purely intrapsychic. This contention would hold that autonomy, or decision making, is also subjective and not observable therefore. In short, it is argued that human b ehavior cannot be measured. I suggest that, on the contrary, autonomy *is* measurable. An infant sucking at the breast "intends" to get fed. Perhaps "intends" is too strong a word; the infant's reasoning and decision-making capacities are undeveloped. Autonomy is more evident during the terrible twos. Here, will, intent and deci-

sion making is only too evident to the mother struggling to control the child. The child clearly intends to control its own behavior and will struggle to do so to the death, so to speak, or to the mother's death if she feels she must win these battles. The point is, such wars are observable and even measurable to onlookers.

Chapter Nine

Physiology of Autonomy: Control of Energy.

Human behavior is controlled energy. The nervous system and the ego which governs it represent a mechanism to control energy. The energy comes from the sun as electromagnetic waves which are collected and stored by the biomass and ingested by humans as food. This in turn is metabolized into glucose, oxidized into adenosine triphosphate which breaks down into adenosine biphosphate, releasing electrons thereby. These energize myofibrils to produce the contraction of smooth and striped musculature which in turn impel movement—action. The nervous system senses food and other humans in the environment and the ego directs the instinctual forces of hunger and social interaction to obtain them. It senses danger and directs the forces of fear and anger to deal with it.

A normal adult is autonomous, He controls his energy—directs his behavior—to survive and procreate. To preserve his "self," he adapts. Inability to do so,the dependence on others for direction, is abnormal.

Although developed psychosocially, this theory of autonomy turns out to have a neuro-physiological basis. When the neurosurgeon Wilder Penfield[45] electrically stimulated a site on a man's motor cortex, the man's arm was elevated. Surprised, the man said, "I didn't do that, you did it." The neuro-electrical circuits of the man's ego, presumably in the prefrontal cortex, had been by-passed anatomically. When a patient, Leslie, assaulted a nurse and then denied doing so, the circuits of her ego had been by-passed psychologically. Since the act of assaulting a nurse was unacceptable to her, she had repressed her ego involvement.

Autonomy depends on the prefrontal cortex—ego functions. The prefrontal area is weak in children and adolescents, and is easily "captured" by adults, including parents. It also weakens in old age and at any age in the presence of prefrontal cortical damage. This makes people dependent on their surroundings with loss of autonomy. It can lead to mimicry, copy-cat behavior, and "madness" [L'hermitte, op.cit. 46]. The prefrontal cortex has a particularly important role in storing the abstract plans and pieces of information used as command signals to carry out the neural work of complex task performance.[47]

The second factor which supports the importance of autonomy is that it depends to some extent on the brain's capacity to inhibit and filter out irrelevant information. The inhibitory system is both cortical and subcortical and is assisted by neurotransmitters. To be in control means that what is now called the "executive cortex" can control input whether from lower, more primitive levels of phylogenetic development, e.g. the limbic system, autonomous from the id, and external stimuli[48].

The enigma of biologic life, particularly of the human mind and consciousness, has been considered beyond the capacity of human intelligence to resolve, and has challenged and baffled mankind since the beginning of time.The nature of human energy remains unstated and unexplained."Drive," "urge," "instinctual energy" are terms used commonly in this respect, but these leave unanswered the question of what is a drive? Or what is the power of an urge?

Treating psychotic patients, I came upon the idea that

humans are controlled by attraction and repulsion, as is elecro-magnetic energy. An argument supporting this notion is that only three forces exist in the universe: the "short force" holding atomic nuclei together, gravity, and electro-magnetic force. Biologic force cannot be either of the first two, so it must be the latter. No one knows what energy is, but that it causes motion and heat is known. Also, the laws which govern electromagnetic energy are well known. So I suggest life is controlled by the laws which govern electromagnetic energy, namely, attraction and repulsion, positive and negative. The most obvious, but naive way to equate positive-negative is with pleasure-pain, or with reward and punishment, or repetition and avoidance. Freud said all behavior is controlled by pleasure and pain. And twenty years ago Olds[op.cit] discovered the "brain reward system" which has now been shown to constitute a major anatomic and physiologic part of the human brain.

The implications of the idea that life is electromagnetic energy are mind-boggling, chiefly because it suggests a way to control a person's behavior. Stated in its simplest terms it states, merely, that a person does, or tries to do, whatever makes him feel good. This hardly appears mind-boggling, rather a truism. But when "feeling good" is understood to have an anatomic physiological basis in the brain, the idea of doing what makes a person feel good begins to be interesting, rather than a truism.

A rat presses a lever wired to reward centers in its brain. The rat does so because it thereby gains "pleasure." I suggest psychological stimuli also may stimulate reward centers in the brain, just as does pressing a wired lever. For example, a person asks a question. Doing so is equivalent to pressing a lever. The sound of the question goes to the recipient who answers. The answer goes to ears of the person who asked the question and thence along auditory pathways of his brain to his reward centers.

Success treating psychotic patients has shown that psychosocially rewarding their autonomous behavior cures these patients. The physician, interacting with the patient, sees what response the patient is trying to elicit and responds so as to make the attempt successful—rewarding. From insane the patients become sane, able to anticipate the effects of their actions and develop adaptive behavior patterns, change from helpless, dangerous patients who have to be controlled and taken care of to responsible citizens living independently.

It is known that dopamine both regulates symptomatology and is a key element of the brain reward system. Creese, Burt and Snyder in 1976[49], showed that schizophrenia represents deficient dopamine transmission, and can be cured by neuroleptics which increase dopamine transmission. This clinical observation suggests that schizophrenia represents a defect in brain reward. My theory suggests that schizophrenia can be cured by psychosocial interaction, which increases dopamine transmission using the brain reward system.

Neuroscience has made enormous and exciting advances in the last twenty-nine years. For example, Heilman, in a single recent article, "The Neurobiology of Emotion,"[50], cites eighty-four references. Neurologic mechanisms of attention, arousal, motor activation are dealt with at length. Positive-negative; pleasure-unpleasure; reward-punishment; anger-fear, are concepts said to explain much neural function. "The cortex is critical in regulating the activities of the limbic system, basal ganglia and reticular system: the left hemisphere mediates positive emotions, the right, negative emotions . . . the right hemisphere is also critical in motor activation."

Although the psychological theory I suggest has a neurophysiological basis, neuroscience has not proposed a corresponding coherent theory of psychological function based on neurophysiological knowledge: no suggestions for treatment of psychopathology, for example, or for resolution of interpersonal conflicts, or for child rearing.

An unresolved problem is that biologic energy is electrochemical, as contrasted to electromagnetic. How to transpose from one to the other? How about tropisms, as in the geotropic nematode worm which crawls up away from gravity—what neural mechanism controls its crawling? The energy involved must be electromagnetic, positive and negative, repulsion and attraction. Could it be pleasure and pain? Could a worm experience pleasure and pain? How about the ciliary movement of a paramecium? This, too, must be energized by electromagnetism. Could it be called pleasure and pain? My suggestion is that biologic energy is controlled by the laws of electromagnetism, whether in complex organisms like humans or relatively simple ones like protozoa.

The inhibitory system of the executive cortex can exclude input of information from the environment or from lower centers of the limbic system. But how does inhibition work? Could it work by positive-negative control? Electrons (-) and protons (+). These questions certainly are beyond my expertise. The notion that tropisms and taxes are controlled or operated by pleasure-pain seems a plausible possibility, and that positive-negative could be so equated.

Humans are binary. Even the information in DNA is digital Almost all words in the English language which refer to human motivation come in dichotomies: yes/no, stop/go, pleasure/ pain, fight/flight, love/hate, good/bad, virtue/evil, succeed/ fail, up/down, strong/weak, smart/dumb, etc. And, as suggested above, all these words operate by underlying reward/punishment, pain/pleasure. It will be argued that humans are too complicated to be governed by + and -, too complicated to be binary. However, computers are complicated, yet they are binary, operate by +, -; or 0, 1. Are humans just a bunch of electric switches? How about God? What does he, or she, have to do with switches? Well, he-she invented the whole arrangement and likes to do things simply: Heaven/Hell, God/Satan.

Epilogue

My theory of autonomy and mental disorder either "attracts, or repels" the reader. In any case, I believe it merits further clinical and neurophysiological testing.

References

1. Lorenz, Konrad Z., *King Solomon's Ring*, New York, Thomas Cowell Co. 1952.

2. Tinbergen, Niko, *The Study of Instinct*, Oxford, Clarendon Press., 1953.

3. Thorpe, William Homan, *Learning and Instinct in Animals,* Harvard University Press, 1956.

4. Wilson, Edward O., *On Human Nature*, Harvard University Press. Cambridge Mass., 1978.

5. Hollobler, Bert and Wilson, Edward O., *Journey to the Ants,* Preface, page ii, Harvard Univ. Press, 1994.

6. American Psychiatric Association, *Diagnostic and Statistical Manual.*, 4th Ed., 1995.

7. Beebe, Gilbert, W. and Appel, John W., *Variation in Psychological Tolerance to Ground Combat in World WarII,* National Academy of Sciences Final Report, #49-007-MD-172. 2101, National Research Council, Division Medical Science., Constitution Ave NW, Washington, DC, 1958.

8. Shurley, Jay T., *Stress and Adaptation as related to sensory/perceptual isolation research,* Military Medicine., 131(3): 254-258, March, 1996.

9. Cannon Walter B., *Bodily Changes in Pain, Hunger, Fear and Rage*, Boston, 1932.

10. Shapiro, David, *Autonomy and Rigid Character*, Basic Books, Inc. New York, 1987.
11. Sullivan, Harry Stack, *The Interpersonal Theory of Psychiatry*, Univ. of Chicago Press, 1950.
12. Burness and Moore, *Compendium of Standard Terms and Concepts of the American Psychoanalytic Association*, Yale University Press, 1995.
13. Fromm-Reichman, Frieda, *Principles of Intensive Psychotherapy*, Univ. of Chicago Press, 1950.
14. Arieti, Silvano, *Interpretation of Schizophrenia*, 2nd Edition., Basic Books, New York, 1974.
15. Rattigan, Terence, *Separate Tales: Two Plays*, Random House, New York, 1957.
16. Marquand, John P. *The Late George Apley* Little Brown, Boston, 1937.
17. Alexander, Franz, *Fundamentals of Psychoanalysis*, 2nd Edition, W.W. Norton, New York, 1948.
18.Erickson, Erick, *Childhood and Society*, 2nd. Edition, Norton, New York, 1963.
19. Kohut, Heinz, *The Analysis of the Sell* University Press, New York, 1971.
20. Mahler, Margaret; Pine, Fred; Bergman, *The Psychological Birth of the Human Infant* Basic Books, Inc. New York, 1975.
21. Piaget, Jean, *Science of Education and the Psychology of the Child*, Orion Press, 1970.
22. Gardner, Howard, *The Unschooled Mind*, Basic Books, 1991.
23. Searle, John. *Mind, Brains and Science*, Harvard Univ. Press, 1984.
24. Rangell, Leo, *Action Theory Within the Structural View*, International Journal of Psychoanalysis, 1989, pg. 189.

25. Fairbairn, W.R.D, *An Object-Relations Theory*, Ed., Jeremy Hazell, 1994.
26. Guntrip, Harry A., *Personal Relations Theory*, Ed., 1994.
27. Bowlby, John, *Secure Base: Parent-Child Attachment and Healthy Development*, 1988.
28. Hartmann, Heinz, *Ego Psychology and the Problem of Adaptation*, International Universities Press, New York, 1939-58.
29. Holt, Robert R., *Autonomy Re-Evaluated*, International Journal of Psychoanalysis, Vol. 3, Jan-June, 1964.
30. Lichtenstein, Heinz, *The Dilemma of Human Identity*, J. Aronson, 1983.
31. Huizenga, Judith, N., Mack, John E. Ed. *Self Esteem and Narcissism, Self Esteem*, International Universities Press New York, 1983, Pgs 151-176.
32. Givelber, Frances. *In Mack*, op. cit.
33. Schafer, Roy. *Retelling a Life*, Basic Books, 1992.
34. Sutherland, John, *The Autonomous Self*, The Work of John Sutherland, Schariff, Jill Sevedge, Ed.
35. Mitchell, Stephen A., *Influence and Autonomy in Psychoanalysis*, The Analytic Press, 1997.
36. Levy, David Mordiceai, *Opposition Syndromes and Oppositional: Behavior in Psychopathology of Childhood*, ed. by Hoch and Zubin, Grune an tratton, New York, pg. 204, 1955.
37. Mahler, Margaret., op. cit.
38. L'Hermitte, F., et al., *Autonomy and the Frontal Lobes Imitation and Utilization Behavior A Neuropsychological Study of 75 Patients*, Annals of Neurology 19, pg 324-336 1986.
39. Routenberg, Aryeh, *The Reward System of the Brain*, The Workings of the Brain. Linas, Rudolfo, Ed. W.H. Freeman N.Y. 1978.

40. Birdwhistell, Ray, *Kinesthetic and Content,* University of Pennsylvania Press, 1971.

41. Darwin, Charles, *The Expression of Emotions in a Man and Animals,* New York University Press, 1969.

42. Phelps, Charlotte, Professor of Economics Temple University. Personal Communication.

43. Lidz, Theodore, *The Origin and Treatment of Schizophrenic Disorders,* New York, Basic Books.

44. Knapp, Peter. Somatization in Burness and Moore, op.cit.

45. Penfield, Wilder, *The Cerebral Cortex of Man, A Clinical Study of Localization of Function,* 1957.

46. L'Hermitte, F. et al. *Autonomy and the Frontal Lobes. Imitation and Utilization Behavior: A Neuropsychological Study of 75 Patients.* Annals of Neurology, 1986, 19, 324-333.

47. Heath, Robt G., *Modulation of Emotion with a Brain Peacemaker,* Journal of Nervous and Mental Disease, 1987, Vol. 165 no. 5.

48. Elliott, Frank T. Professor of Neurology, University of Pennsylvania. Personal Communication.

49. Creese, Ian; Burt, R. David, and Snyder, Solomon H. *Dopamine Receptor Binding Predicts Clinical and Pharmacological Pontencies of Anti-Schizophrenic Drugs, Science,* April Vol. 2 Spring pg 481-483 1976. Alos see Neland C. Tomas, *Pathopsychology of Schizophrenia: Dopamine Hypothesis,* American Journal of Neuropsychiaty Vol. 8, Number 2, Spring 1996.

50. Heilman, Kenneth M. *The Neurobiology of Emotional Experience.* Journal of Neuropsychiatry, Vol. 9., Number 3, Summer, 1997.